Hi!

Welcome to the pole comr

Now that you're here, I hear you ask: 'Where do I start?'

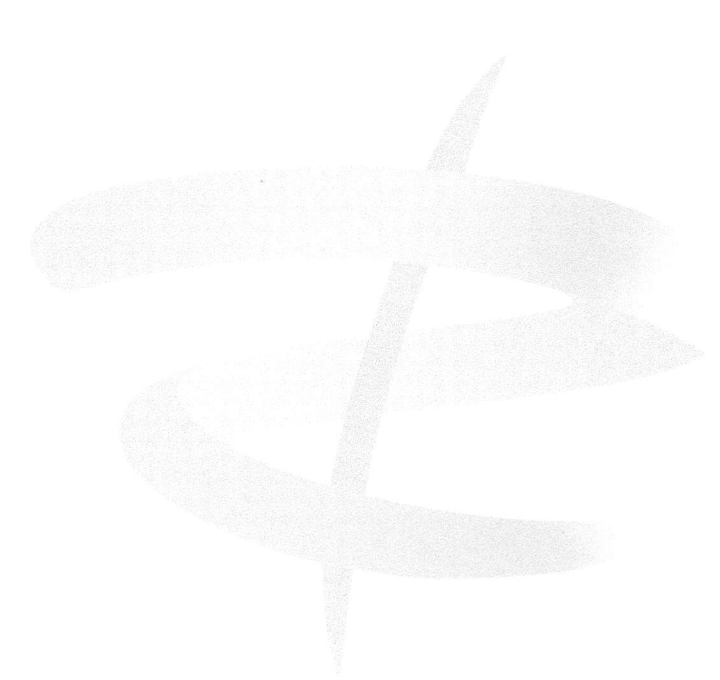

You're here, you're excited, and you've got the pole, but holy moly! The moves you find online that people say are for beginners—it's bonkers! And honestly, it's unsafe. The industry has grown so much over the last 2 decades, and what used to be advanced is old news, having somehow become beginner level.

As we've all gotten older, we've forgotten where we started. The journey has been lost. Have a few children, and by George, you remember! Some of the intense moves I still had, but the so-called easy ones? Lost in space!

I sat down and worked it out, step by step, muscle by muscle, move by move. And now I'm here to share that with you. Why? Because I love pole. I love the sense of constant achievement. Each move is a goal, and each goal achieved makes you feel amazing. Suddenly, you're doing things you never thought possible. You had no idea that move was what you were working up to! I love helping people grow, do things they didn't think they could, and achieve the feeling of empowerment that comes with this. I don't want people getting injured on the way by not knowing their path. The journey is ahead, and this is your first step.

Please be aware: this book is only a guide. There is a huge range of moves you can do from each of those I have given you. Everyone's body is different, and as much as pole doesn't discriminate against gender, body type, or anything like that, adjustments can be made to suit you.

Training from home is fantastic – you're not as self-conscious – but you also don't have that 'Wow! They're the same as me; I'm doing okay, then!' or 'Look at that! I must try that!' reaction. Training buddies are good value and good inspiration! There's so much value in going to a studio and having an instructor point out if your hips or shoulders aren't square, remind you to pull more with your top arm, or tell you to bring your bottom arm down a little more. All those little tips that come with experience are so helpful.

I understand that studio access isn't always possible. I have lived hours away from the closest pole studio; I started teaching at midnight in my tin shed to escape the heat! Sometimes, options aren't available. I just want you to be safe and to have an understanding of the path to pole glory! Remember, it is a high-risk sport. Look after your body. Warm up, cool down, use a crash mat, and if you have a spotter, use them when you're trying a new high-risk move. However, don't think of a crash mat as a safe zone and allow yourself to fall. If you're unsure if you're ready to do the move, more preparation is needed! But when you are ready, have your crash mat ready, just to be sure. Stay safe!

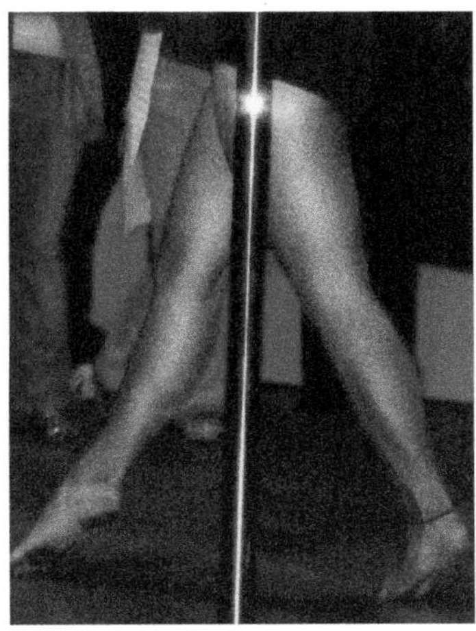

Disclaimer:

I'm a pole fitness instructor and not a healthcare professional. This book only provides general information about pole fitness and does not consider your personal circumstances in any way. Pole Fitness is a high-risk sport. You should consult your health care professional before starting any fitness program to ensure that it is right for your needs and abilities. Do not start a pole fitness program if your pole fitness instructor or health care provider advises against it. Please monitor and work within your own limitations, and stop immediately if you experience things like faintness, dizziness, pain, or even shortness of breath at any time while exercising. Remember that your body needs to rest. Training regimes need to allow for rest and recovery as well. This guide is not a substitute for skilled instruction. We recommend seeking professional instruction from a pole fitness instructor before attempting a pole fitness program on your own, always having competent individual close by to assist if needed. Please ensure that your pole set-up and area is secure, safe and as per manufactures specifications, ensuring an unobstructed space. To the extent permitted by law, I disclaim any liability (including in negligence) arising directly or indirectly from your use of the information contained in this book.

Any reference to treatments, wives' tales remedies or other recommendations are only for interest and need to be followed up with a healthcare practitioner prior to considering implementing them. Following any advice in this book is at your own risk. Rapture Arts or any of the contributors in this book cannot be held liable for your actions after reading the book.

I'm totally proud of this book!

I have a few people to thank for helping make it a reality.

Cover photography: © Jealous by Nature

(You guys are amazing!)

*Photo taken in Margaret River, Western Australia.

Sketch animation artwork: © Gavin Hunter from Wild Body Art

(Thank you for making my little details come to life!)

The amazing anatomy artwork: © Slaybaugh Studios – you're amazing Tiffany!!

And to all the people who gave never-ending feedback on design as we went. You guys are superb! To Joanna, Neo, Danielle, Kelly, Cameron, and Mum, thank you for helping me put together and create the whole package.

My husband: I totally sprang this book on you, announcing not only that I was going to write a book but that I had almost finished one! You have supported me through every step of this journey. Together, we make it an adventure. Thank you. (And thank you for picking up the camera when I asked you to take the photos I needed!)

My students: you are my inspiration. Watching you grow and growing with you has been a very special journey. Thank you!

And the kids: like, wow. Writing a book with young kids in the house, somehow, we made it work. My amazings, you really are super special! Your pole journey started young, and your strength is inspiring to so many. I hope this book inspires you. Follow your dreams, my darlings!

To you, reader, this book is for you. Thank you for allowing me to be part of your adventure. May you have a safe journey through the world of pole fitness. May it inspire and empower not only you but those around you.

Enjoy the journey!

Lara xx

Lara xxx

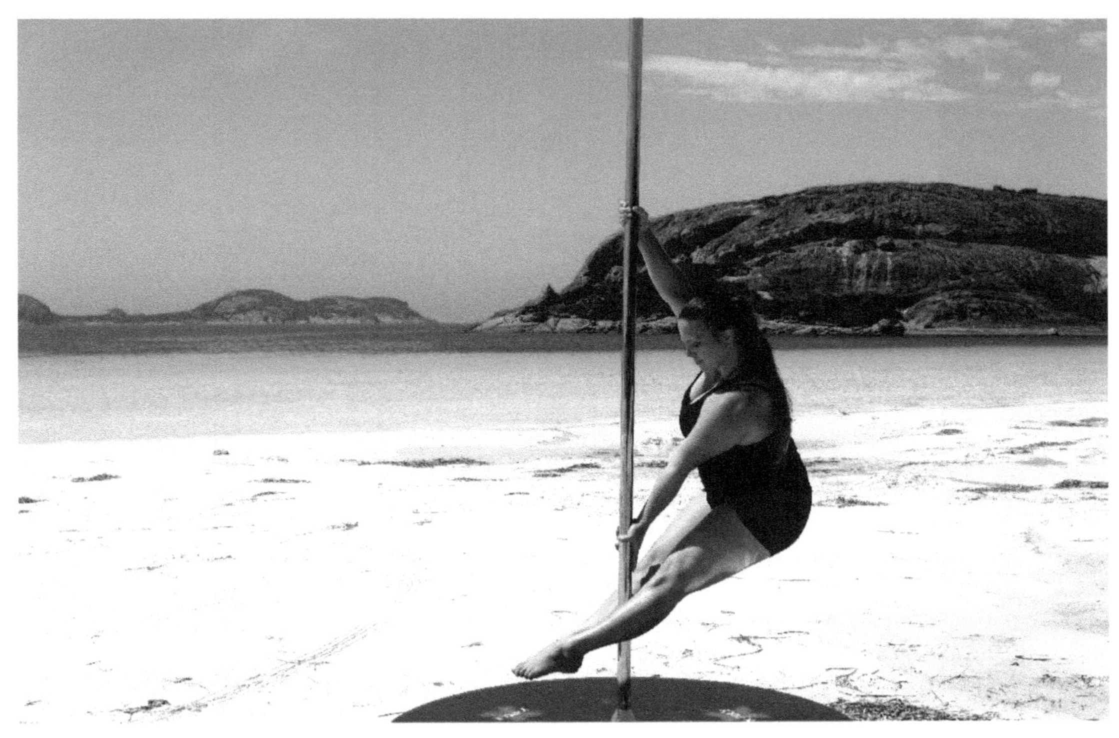

First paperback edition July 2021

ISBN: 978-0-6450176-0-1

eBook ISBN: 978-0-6450176-1-8

Table of Contents

About the Author

Lara Johnson started learning pole fitness in 2006. She loved the sense of achievement and empowerment she got from achieving new tricks, and by 2007, she was teaching and performing in Perth, Western Australia.

She travelled around Australia to attend workshops, learning from the best in the fields of circus and pole fitness. Lara has now taught all around Western Australia, working alongside some amazing artists.

Lara's drive to understand how moves work led her to study fitness (Certificate III and IV). Over 10 years later, she obtained international certification to teach pole dance (IPDFA), and she trained in aerial yoga instruction.

Lara has also taught and performed lyra and other circus acts, including aerials at camps and shows in Western Australia and along Australia's east coast. Lara spent many years working at team-building camps for the State Government, which cemented her love of helping people achieve new goals.

After slowing down to start her family, in 2017, Lara moved to Margaret River and set up a pole fitness studio called Rapture Arts. There, she shares a sense of achievement and empowerment and the gift of flight with her students.

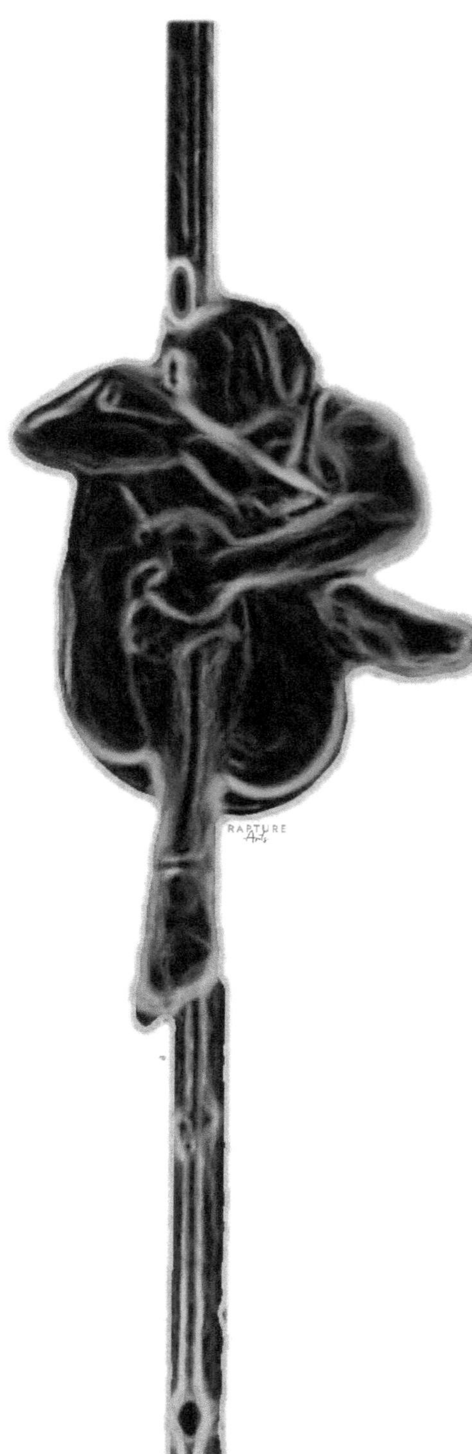

Learning the Technical Stuff

Pole fitness is fun! If you go to gentleman's clubs and see the girls who make a living there, you'll notice that many don't even take their feet off the floor! You could do a whole session (or even a course!) on sensual movement. There are many styles of pole dance. You can adjust it to your level and your goals and take it as far as you like. You don't need to go upside down or up the pole; you can stay with low-flow moves or go an acrobatic route with flips and jumps. Whatever your style or goal, we all start somewhere.

The list of pole spins is ridiculous, and these can help you gain grip and arm, shoulder, and core strength. From there, you'll have the strength to progress up the pole. Once comfortable at a height, you can invert. That's 3 steps right there, with many weeks, even months, spent on each. And there are more steps after inverting! Eek!

Eventually, pole dancing is quite a high-risk activity, but if you progress slowly, moving through each stage, not only will your strength solidify and stabilise, but your understanding of how your body works around the pole will grow. This will turn going upside down into a manageable and lower-risk affair! Don't let this scare you away. You can go as far as you are comfortable and maintain awareness of your body and your personal limits. There's so much you can do and learn without going to the extreme.

So, you're standing there, looking at your pole. You've set it up like the book said, whether it's on the rafters or freestanding. You've seen all the internet fails and don't want to be next! You've followed the manufacturer's instructions – tension checked (double-checked, maybe triple-checked). Yep, that thing is stuck!

But before, it was shiny, and now there are smudge marks all over it. Those smudge marks are the natural oils from your skin. It happens, so don't stress. However, it does add to slipperiness, especially if you moisturised this morning. I got into the habit of moisturising at night and using a makeup brush to put moisturiser on in the morning (until I found a face one that didn't add to my slip!) Ironically, if your skin gets too dry, it also makes the pole slippery; the balancing act of each individual skin type begins! Avoid oil-based products. I've heard that glycerine-based products can be

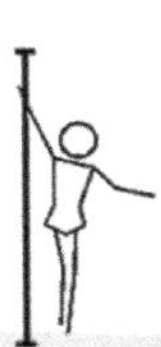

very effective for some dry-skin polers who need to moisturise, while others use aloe vera, but you'd need to do a test patch; always try new products carefully.

Back to those smudge marks. Grab a flannel and a smidgen of water, and wipe them off. Done! I clean with methylated spirits before and after each training session but just use a damp cloth during training, sometimes soapy water, depending on the day. Some days I wipe the pole once or twice during training, other days after every move. Flow with it, but also have fun with it. Think of cleaning the pole as part of the 'act' if you were on stage, everyone would see you clean the pole, it isn't a chore, it is all part of the act. Play it, make the most of it, enjoy how you can move, as you clean the pole.

You'll notice that each day, each season, your grip changes, depending on the humidity and moisture in the air, on the temperature, on your skin grip – all sorts. Learn to work with it. A move that you use one day may not be worth training another. Otherwise, clean down the pole every 5 seconds.

I warm up and stretch on the pole prior to every training session. It gives my skin a chance to adjust and gives me a chance to see how slippery the day is. Plus, it warms the cold pole up! I'd recommend not fighting slippery days. If you can find a way to balance it, fab! If not, train pole moves that take you to the ground, like floorwork and transitions from floor to standing. Practise getting stuck on your bottom with the pole between your legs, and work out creative ways out. Listen to music, and move around the pole, getting lost in the lyrics and movement.

Grip can suck, but there are options! Back in the old days, no one in my class used anything. We gained strength and found that our grip adjusted with time. I never jumped onto a smaller pole, as I found I had grip on a 50 mm pole, not a 45 mm pole. On the odd occasion, I heard I should try hair spray for grip. Then came all these products.

Yes, they all have their advantages and disadvantages, and each one is made for a different skin type. But at $20 for a little bottle, it's up to you if it's the path you want to take. Initially, however, you want to get used to your grip and gain strength without relying on product. Products may change your body's responses. If you're sweaty, it's probably for a reason. It could be nerves or something else. Using a product to dry out your skin can sometimes make your body produce more sweat in the end, creating a vicious cycle and a reliance on the product. Starting without grip aids allows your body to adjust, then hopefully not need a product at all.

The cheap way out, if you want to purchase something, one option is non-moisturising shaving cream. It gives you a bit of tack if your skin is on the dry side. However, many people find that it increases the slip, you also need to consider skin sensitivities. If your skin is prone to being more slippery and sweaty, soapy water works just as well. But like I said, learn without product. Chances are, you won't need it. I have a damp cloth, which I use to wipe down the pole and my hands during each training session as needed as my skin is on the dryer side. If you get to elaborate inversions, you can decide then, once you have strength and knowledge of your grip and how your body works with the apparatus.

In saying all this, there are always exceptions. Some people may have super strong hands and amazing grip capability but also amazing slip. This is okay. It's just your body type. Now it's a case of finding the right product, if any, to assist you in your journey.

Grip Strengthening

Grip strengthening is also a thing. Your hands are what are looking after you, so you also need to spend a bit of time looking after them! Not just strengthening them, but also warming them up and preparing them for exercise. There are many ways to approach grip strength. I used to sit on a bus and flick my fingers out as fast and wide as I could, then curl them back into a fist and flick them out again and again and again. This is an awesome move for grip strength.

Something as simple as squeezing a stress ball – squeeze, hold, and release – can help. The softer the ball, the easier it is, so if it's too easy, slowly work up to a tennis-ball type item.

Whether you have kids or not, just hanging on the monkey bars is good. To make it more dynamic, swing your way across the bars, either with your palms facing away from you in the middle rungs or with your palms facing each other on the outer supporting bars. This gets your wrists working at different angles to support your grip.

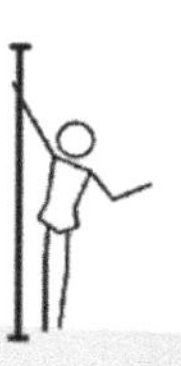

You can also do simple movements on the floor from kneeling. Lay your hands flat on the floor, then lift your palms and place them back down, repeating this.

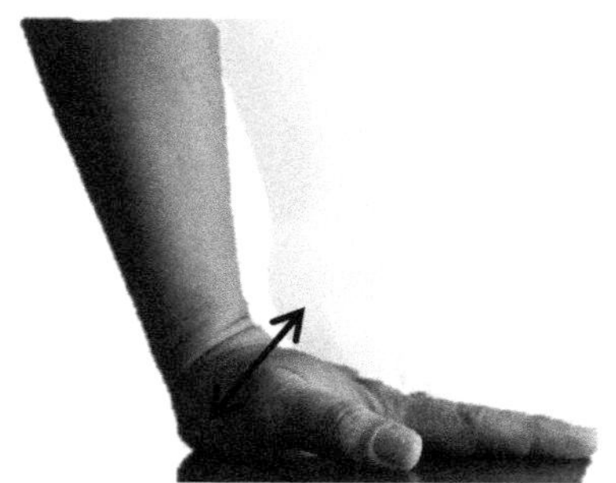

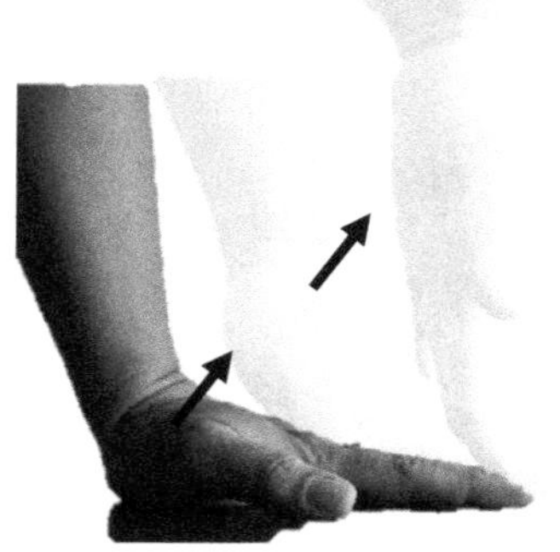

The next step is to break that into 2. Lift your palms off the floor, then up onto the tips of your middle 3 fingers. Place your fingers back down on the floor, followed by your palm.

A really strange-feeling strengthening technique involves creating a fist with your thumb on the outside. With your hands facing inward and the flat punching end of your fists on the floor in front of you, rock forward onto them. Next, rotate your fist forward so that the circle your hand and thumb create touches the ground. Then rock back onto the punching part of your fist. Remember, use small, slow, controlled movements. Don't rush!

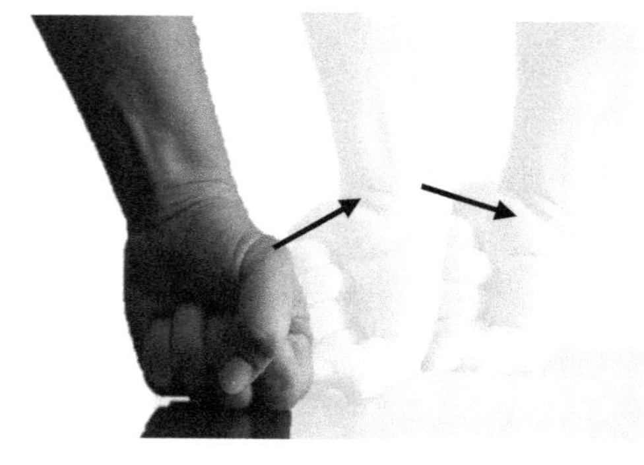

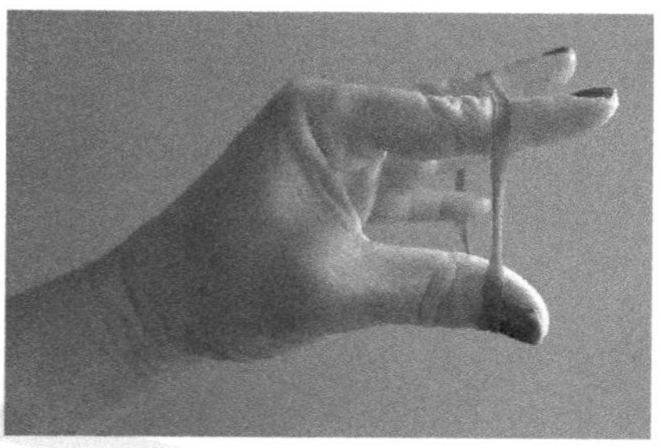

If you want to intensify your grip training, pop an elastic band around your fingertips while they're in a hand puppet position (thumb and fingers together). Practise opening your fingers out and controlling them as you close them again. If the elastic band is too loose, wrap it around a second time, but make sure it's not so tight that you stress about circulation.

Carrying things around the house is also a good way to strengthen grip. Grab a book or something that won't break or get damaged if dropped. Place your fingers on one side and your thumb on the other. Let the item hang beside you, and carry it around.

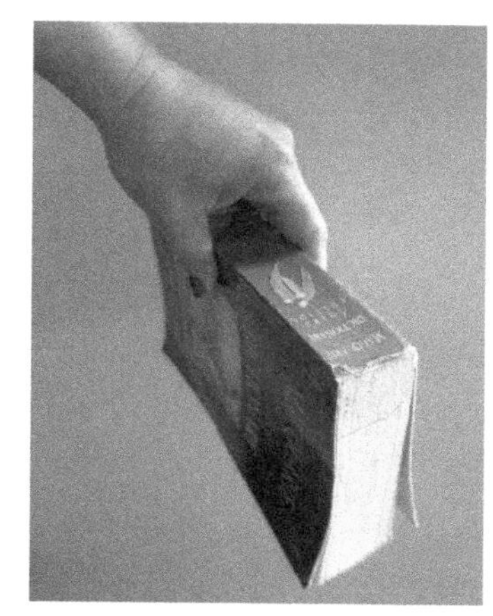

Again, if you have kids, playdough uses all sorts of muscles. When I hurt my hand and was starting the journey to restrengthen it, my specialist got me to play with plasticine and playdough. I also had to open and close my hand in a bag of rice so that there was resistance all around it. It's funny the things you can come up with to make training a bit of an adventure! You could bake some bread from scratch one day, and hey presto! All that kneading is conditioning with a warm treat at the end of it.

One thing that's often forgotten with grip is to include hand/finger stretching in your warm-up/stretch routine. Finger flicks are great. Flicking your fingers out as far and fast as you can. You can also make your hands into a puppet, like you're doing the chicken dance or being a snake, and make the puppet talk. (Yep! I like to make warm-ups interesting!) Having a flat hand and spreading your fingers apart before bringing them back together is also really good. Handshakes and forearm stretches can allow you to lead these movements on to the rest of the body and create your own rotation of stretches and warm-ups. This helps your grip strength, and as your hands are literally holding you, you want to look after them. Make sure not to forget about them!

Jewellery

Jewellery looks beautiful. It's sentimental, and sometimes, it doesn't feel right to take it off. But rings can scratch your pole. I also find they hinder my grip; I always feel more slippery when I forget to take my rings off. Watches and bracelets can get in the way of the movement in your wrist. And necklaces? If you're upside down, they're in your face, and the last thing you want is for your necklace to get caught while it's around your neck. It's best to remove all jewellery for safety's sake.

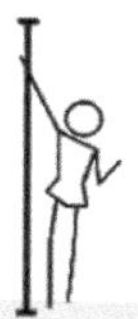

Move Variations

Please remember that everyone's body is different. Some people have short arms, while others have long arms. There are differences in torso length and width, bust size, flexibility, joint mobility – everything! Moves can be adjusted.

Can't get your outside arm across your chest to the pole? Change the angle of your body to the pole. Maybe step back from the pole, or stand closer to bring your outside hand up higher, like you're holding a baseball bat. Or slide your outside arm directly under your chest. Alternatively, try another grip. Maybe one day, once you have stable shoulder muscles and activation, you'll favour one-handed spins. Needless to say, there are options!

Some people have gaps between their thighs, which can hinder some moves. Others have thighs that prevent their feet from coming together, which can hinder other moves. Each person has their strengths. You just need to work on and focus on your strengths and style. I find that I have to lean out to get my bust around the pole sometimes, while others may find their bust completely hindering. If angle changes don't work, try grip changes, always ensuring that you have correct alignment and muscle activation.

There are so many variations for each move, so don't get stuck on a move if your body won't allow it. See what options are out there to safely adjust the move, finding a way to work with your strengths.

Taking photos is a really good habit to get into. Mostly for the purpose of motivation and direction. It is not unusual to forget what you have been training, especially if training the many variations of moves. Photos mean you can create your own record of your training, like your own personal pole-moves' directory. But also mean that you can see the shape you create, are your toes pointed, how do the lines and angles in your body look? These give you pointers on what to work on next. They also over time show how much you've grown on your journey, and if you have an unmotivated day, it can help lift your spirits seeing that you have progressed. Whether that be in moves and levels, or in pointed toes and straight legs. Little Videos also help you see transitions; entries and exits in your moves. Which allow you to plan your training and aid in your progressions.

Defining Pole Types

'I just kind of picked my pole.' But did you really know what you were looking at? The variety of poles these days is amazing. There are stainless steel poles, silicone poles, brass poles, powder-coated poles, and more. And then there are different widths. There are located, fully removable, and freestanding poles. Technical talk much! Here's a brief rundown.

Permanent

Permanent poles are bolted to the ceiling and floor. They're perfect for higher ceilings, as they're sturdy and can support heavier loads. However, you can't just pack them away, and there will always be permanent markings on the ceiling.

Semi-permanent (or located)

Semi-permanent are sort of a mix of the permanent poles. They're still fixed to the ceiling with permanent brackets. However, these poles can be removed from their brackets to allow the space to be used for something else. This generally limits the height of your pole, as you can only go as high as your space. Semi-permanent poles are fine for houses, raised ceilings, and all that jazz.

Friction/jacked poles (or fully removable)

Friction/jacked poles do not bolt to the ceiling or floor. Some appear to have what looks like a suction cup on the top, while others appear to have a wide rubber ring. These poles have an internal spring-loaded mechanism that applies outward pressure, and this pressure is distributed to the wide discs at the top and bottom of the pole.

You always need to ensure you get the right-sized pole for your space and that you put your pole on the supporting beam in your roof. Otherwise, it may crack the ceiling. These poles have limitations with regard to their stability and load, so it's important to not forgo quality. Cheapies may not actually be metal on the inside.

Generally, these poles come with the ability to be stationary or to spin and are reasonably easy to set up and move. Personally, though, I'd prefer to set my pole up properly once and not have to move it again! These poles must be set up and aligned right. They can produce scuff marks when removed, but once removed, they can be stored quite compactly.

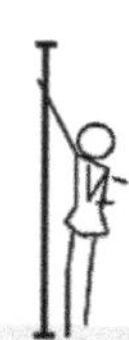

Portable poles

Portable poles are similar to friction/jacked poles. Make sure you have a reputable brand. These poles are made for easy dismantling and storage, but I'd be wary of something made to be taken down easily, as it must be sturdy enough for use.

Stage/freestanding poles

These poles are not a cheap option, but if you have a raked ceiling, are wary of putting a pole up in a rental, or want to take your pole out and about, they are a very viable option. These poles do make floorwork a bit more difficult, and you'll need to be aware of your routine so as to avoid falling off the stage or rolling an ankle. You'll also need to be aware of the height of your pole. If you train in heels, is your pole still high enough?

Stage/freestanding poles come with round or square bases. Round bases are more common, with some stages being more compact and transportable than others. Due to there being no top support, the stabilisers are all in the base, which can make it quite heavy. There will also be a natural wobble at the top. Some stage poles need sandbags or extra stabilisers under the stage as well.

These types of poles may need a large vehicle for transport. However, some fold up quite compactly. For my first stage pole, I needed a trailer; the second fits in the back of the car.

Stage/freestanding poles are great for tradeshows and outside displays or high-ceiling presentation nights. They generally come in spinning and static options. There's no need to screw or unscrew anything (generally); it's just a case of piecing it all together. These poles are usually more expensive, as you have to pay for the stage as well, but they may offer the solution you're looking for.

You can also get freestanding poles with a thinner base, which means the pole doesn't go up as high. This makes poles easier to set up and remove, though some people find the height of shorter poles limiting. You can usually purchase adjustments to make your pole fit your space.

Pole construction

Spinning poles

Spin gives a floaty, dramatic influence to your routines, as moves that you'd usually just pose in become fluid and move with you. You can increase and decrease speed using the laws of physics as you go through a routine. Spinning poles are usually used by more experienced dancers, as there is a higher risk of injury. This isn't just due to the spin factor. Spinning can make you feel like you're getting a move right when you're not, and incorrect body alignment isn't good for your muscles and joints.

Spin also encourages you to be one-sided in your training, as you'll naturally stimulate the pole to move in the same direction. Being one-sided isn't good for your muscles and joints either. I've found that many students who train predominantly on spinning poles become one-sided to the point of losing alignment if they aren't careful when on a spinning pole. They also struggle to create a strong, dynamic grip on the pole and have a harder time moving from one pole type to another. It's almost like driving a manual or automatic car. If you got your licence to drive auto, you often won't be able to drive manual.

Spinning poles are also more expensive than their static counterparts due to the extra construction requirements. You can also get poles that are static and spinning. They can be adjusted using an Allen key or a quick-release lock.

Grip is a big thing for dancers who move from static to spinning poles. On a static pole, you have more dynamic movement, so your grip needs to be adjusted accordingly. Your hand grip will be looser to allow for the pole to glide around your hand. On a spinning pole, the spinning hand usually stays in the same position. Yes, a spinning hand is a thing! In upright spins, this is your top hand, leaving you a more free-flowing bottom hand to help with your movement. This will make more sense when you start looking at grip changes and one-handed spins. The top hand is ALWAYS on the pole and really promotes the spin. It's the bottom that you can play with and adjust.

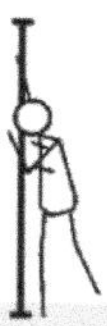

Static poles

Static poles are the best poles to get started on. They give you a chance to orientate yourself around the pole, and they allow you to feel how your body lifts and moves and make adjustments. If you're not rotating or spinning effectively around the pole, you can look at why and work on fixing your posture. This, I find, is one of the best technique fixers. On a static pole, if the move isn't working, you need to fix your technique! You have more control early on with the level of spin that you feel comfortable with.

Static poles require a different, more dynamic level of strength than spinning poles, as you are not only lifting into the position of a spin but are using velocity to create a fluid movement. What may be a conditioning move on a static pole may be a pretty move on a spinning pole, so stylistically, the 2 types can be quite different. Nonetheless, it's best to start on the static. Once you know what you're doing, you can move across and find your own preference.

Thicknesses

Different thicknesses work for different people. The thicker the pole, the more hand strength is needed. The thinner the pole, the more you can wrap your hand around it. When I started, I trained on a 50 mm pole and loved it! Purely because I felt the need to have something that felt bigger so that I felt that it could support me, whereas really, any of the pole sizes would have. Now the common sizes are 45 mm or 38 mm. The thicker the pole the more grip/hand strength developed. So, it is easier to go from a thicker pole to a thinner one, yet harder to go the other way around.

Thickness is generally a personal preference. Do you want to feel like you're holding on to something substantial that really supports you, or do you want to feel like you're holding on and wrapping your whole hand around the pole?

Some moves, especially leg-gripping moves, will be easier on a thicker pole with more pole to grip. Others will be easier on a thinner pole that you can get your body around more easily. It's totally a personal preference. I've found that people with conditions like arthritis in their hands find thinner poles easier, but everyone is different!

Pole Skin

Stainless Steel

Stainless steel used to be the most common option for studio poles (at least when I started out, they appeared to be). However, there are many options out there these days. Stainless steel has a great grip factor and keeps its shine really well. I struggle with matte (non-shiny) stainless steel poles, as I find them much harder to grip, but it's not impossible.

Brass

Brass is more porous, so it offers a better grip. It does tend to tarnish, but if you polish it, it fills all those little porous holes and makes the pole more slippery, so maintenance is more difficult. Tomato paste does the trick to remove tarnish from brass poles.

Powder Coated

I haven't had much experience with powder-coated poles (I did once try to lock my powder-coated Lyra pole when I don't think it was supposed to and scratching the thing in the process!). These poles from my experience do have good grip, and they allow you to colour code! They also 'warm up' quite quicky, and tend to be the choice for those who find metal poles too slippery. Some people find humidity and sweat working against them with powder coated poles, so do your research for your area/skin type just to be sure it is the right fit for you. I personally, would be aware of chipping a powder coated pole, and if there is a chip, does it affect your spin/grip after, the odd pinch-y spot may be annoying, but if you look after and maintain your poles properly, and as per manufacturers specifications this should not be an issue. I have spoken to many people who have powder coated poles and absolutely love them. Some of which have chips in it, and say that it doesn't affect the performance. The good thing is, that the chips, generally stay just that, there is no extra flakes that come off. Maintenance of the pole is also a bonus in comparison to the brass pole, which is also often picked for its good grip-properties. Please be cautious if you do have a metal allergy, as powder coated poles are metal based.

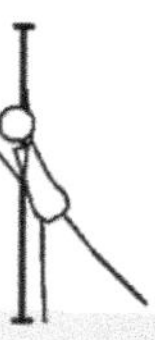

Silicone

Then there's silicone. Honestly, I've never used silicone, but not having to take your trousers off in winter would be amazing, though leggings are still a tad chilly! I have grippy pole trousers for days when it's too cold for shorts. These trousers have their pros and cons, but I'm not sure if the pros and cons of grippy attire would be the same as with a silicone pole, apart from the main one, of grippy attire fashion being predominately female, whereas a silicone pole isn't gender specific. Many people see it as a con to not be able to slide in the grippy trousers, however it does mean that you gain extra control in moves in order to be able to lift and place your limbs onto the pole. In saying this, I predominately use a static pole, and the ability to slide through your hand, and different grip locations becomes a big deal with moves and thus the style of dance would need to change to suit the pole. If your style has more holds, or even more extreme flips, tricks and "power-moves" silicone is a good fit, in this respect it is the dance-pole industries version of Chinese-pole.

Due to the grip-factor, you shouldn't go bare skin on silicone, so these poles may be very similar to Chinese rubber poles, which can cause burns on bare skin. However, that's just speculation from my experience with rubber poles and what I have heard about the "pole kisses" from silicone. Unlike with Chinese rubber poles, where denim trousers and shoes are regularly worn, with silicone, you'll want tight-fitting clothes so you don't slide out of them while up the pole. Many people find it a bonus if uncomfortable, or unable to wear "booty shorts" to train, as it allows different options.

Please note that when it comes to cleaning silicone poles, you'll need a proper silicone cleaner or a similar product as recommended by your pole's manufacturer.

Chrome

Chrome poles are also quite popular; however, I personally find that I slipped more on my chrome than any other pole type. In saying that I know many people who have no issues with Chrome, so this may just be my skin-type. They are popular pole skin for beginners and a pretty good all-rounder pole. Unless a nickel allergy is present, the chrome plating in many brands of poles, does have small traces of nickel which may cause a variety of rashes in those who have allergies- sometimes mistaken for the grip aid reacting, so a process of eliminating one element at a time may be needed to determine if it is a product that you are putting on, or the pole. Also researching the brand that you are looking at purchasing to see if any allergens are present. Chrome poles tend to be more popular in the warmer climates, however I have heard of instances of rust in more humid environments.

Are you itching to get on your pole yet?

We're almost there!

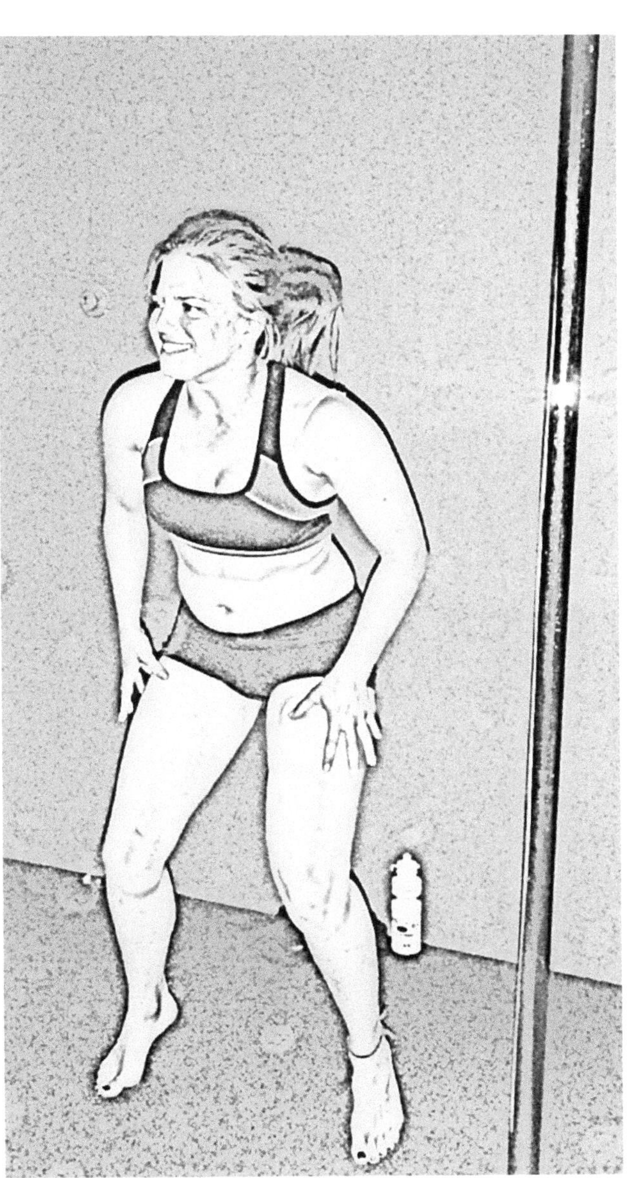

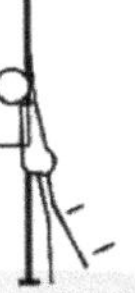

Space Needed

How much space do you need? You learn to work with what you have!

Obviously, try and give yourself space. At the very least, for most moves, a good guide is being able to walk around the pole with an arm out and not touch anything. As moves progress, a 1.5 m radius is a good gauge. But you'll learn where to start a spin, how much momentum to put in, where to land, and which way to face when doing each move.

You'll make it work for your space. If there's a protruding angle, one option is to get a cheap yoga mat and cut it up, attaching it a few folds to the protrusion so that if you do accidentally impact with it, it's not solid wood (or whatever else) that you're kicking. If you can avoid protrusions, awesome. If not, get accustomed to your space and how to move within it. Always being aware of where you are in the space, to avoid them, pets are also a consideration in this regard, it is best to ensure that your pets are not in the room when you are training.

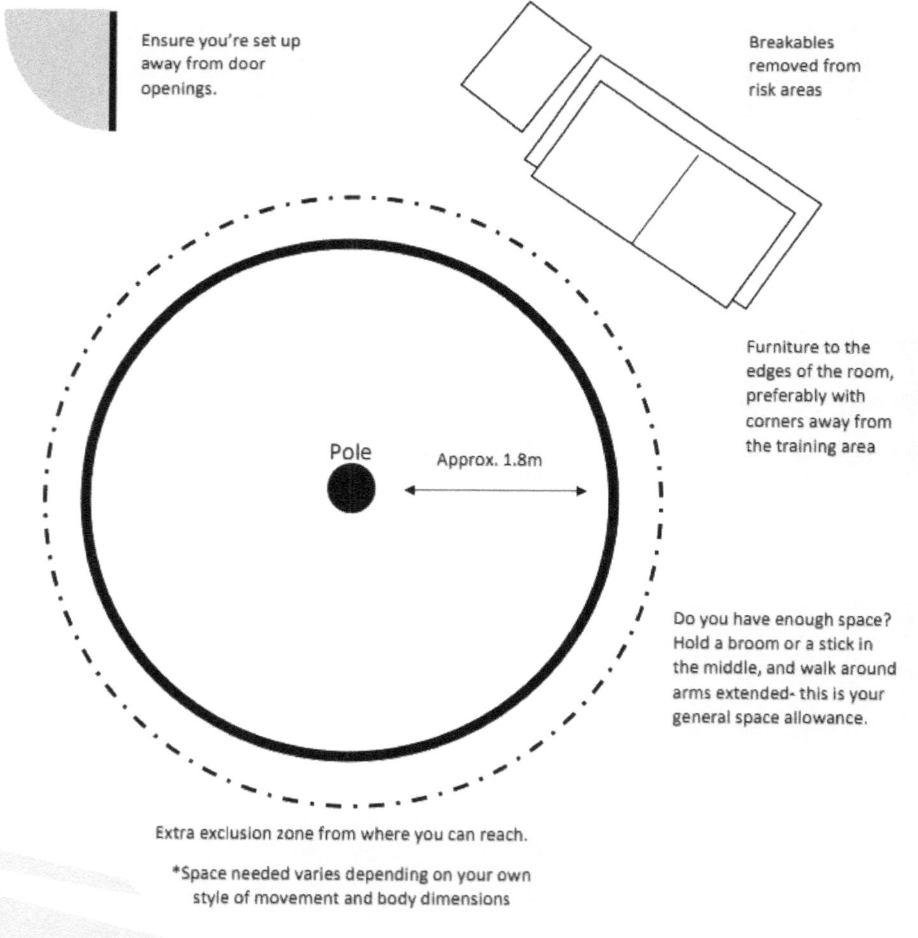

Things that are good to be aware of…

Once you start pole dancing, chances are that you won't want to stop! Pole dancing increases muscle mass and upper body strength and can decrease body fat, as well as improving body image and mental health. The little goals you achieve can really give you a confidence boost!

Once you're in the pole community, you'll realise that judgement of pole dance really comes from the outside.[1] Joanna Nichols did a lot of research on this to find out a bit more about the mental and physical benefits of pole fitness. Following safe practices and progressions during training is shown to grow confidence levels of those participating as well as so many other health and fitness benefits.

So, you get the pole a bit now. One thing you need to be aware of when training is fatigue. It's a thing, and it totally sucks! You get to this point of 'I know I can do this', but it just isn't working. Welcome to fatigue, the doorway to injuries. Listen to your body, and don't push it. When it's done, it's done. Want to keep training? Try different muscle groups, or try floorwork. When I'm feeling fatigued, I often end up doing an awesome stretching session, as that winds me down but makes me still feel productive. That way, I'm satisfied at the end of the session instead of frustrated that my body just isn't working!

It's so important in pole that you listen to your body and adjust for it. If you don't, one day, you might be upside down, and guess what's closest to the floor? Yep, your head! Fatigue is easily recognisable, and you'll notice when it's coming, largely because your body won't let you get into a position it can normally do – very noticeable when it comes to doing more advanced moves, like going upside down. Save yourself, and listen to what your body is saying. Your body will tell you when you still have the strength to get down safely. As long as you always use safe dismounts and avoid dropping out of moves, you should still be able to get down safely from higher-risk moves. As long as you take the cues that your body is giving you, and adjust your training as you notice fatigue coming on.

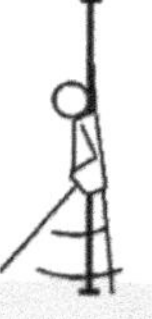

If you're a silly Vegemite and are training with an injury or working outside of your limits and trying things you aren't ready for, that's a completely different kettle of fish. Just don't! Your body is amazing. It can do some splendid things, but it also 'talks' to you. Listen, be nice to it, and train within your personal limits.

Bruises

When I say be nice to your body, I don't mean you're not going to bruise it! Bruises are a part of pole fitness. In fact, they're called 'pole kisses'. Polers often compare bruises and can tell what you've been working on depending on where your bruises are. They even share photos! I love how supportive the pole community is! Yes, bruises are a stage that will come back as you try new things. But eventually, they fade, and you'll be able to spin, sit, and one-leg hang bruise-free! It's just a case of allowing your skin to get accustomed to contact, building your skin's resilience, and allowing it to adjust to the pressure and grip on the pole. Focus on correct posture and technique. Ensuring that you have the correct attachment points with the pole goes a long way.

To start our learning journey of bruises, what comes up, must come down! If you jump up to get onto the pole, you will have that same level of force pulling you down – ouch! Let's not jump. Instead, stabilise, place, and hold. Also, if you slam your leg into the pole, it hurts! Again, take it one step at a time. Place one hand on, followed by the other hand, one leg, and the other leg until you get the hang of it and can play with momentum. Otherwise, a bit of ice and some arnica may go a long way.

I've also heard that butter is amazing for bruises. Keep in mind that if you put it on and then jump on a pole, you'll be in slip central! Wait until you've finished training. For bruising, one of the remedies you hear about most often is arnica. So, what does arnica do? It brings white blood cells[22] to the area and improves circulation, which helps with the bruise factor. It's also said to be an anti-inflammatory and, apparently, a very gentle analgesic. Now, I say this, but science hasn't backed it up. According to a scientific study on the effects of topical arnica on muscle pain, it actually does the opposite, with pain lasting 24 hours longer.[2]

Unfortunately, there haven't been many studies on the effectiveness of arnica in this respect. However, there have been 2 studies of arnica for osteoarthritis. These showed decreased pain with prolonged use, so one would assume that there has to be something helpful in it![3, 4]

So, let's look into bruises a bit. Basically, phosphates make up the blood vessel wall[24]. Skin is full of blood vessels, so the technical side is handy to know. When you give yourself a decent ouch, your body sends histamines to the irritated area[25]. This breaks down cell walls. Are you with me so far? All of a sudden, it's the cell walls of the blood vessels that are damaged, and this causes bleeding into the tissue to form a bruise. [26]

Now there is no scientific research to back this one up, however, butter – not margarine or try-to-be-butter stuff – is supposedly, high in fat and thus, phosphates. The magical big word! Smoosh some butter on your bruise, and help rebuild those damaged cell walls! Or so the theory goes. Makes sense, right? You've got to love *(some)* old wives' tales and remedies! I haven't tried this one, but I have seen people who have the day after they've bonked their head (not from pole), and if there weren't an egg, you'd barely be able to see anything. Mind blown! Butter added to the list of long-lost amazing potential 'remedies'![5] This is the same reason why in old country and Western movies, you see people using steak for bruises: phosphates! There are some people that can get irritations and need to be cautious with phosphates, trying new things should always be approached with caution. Now I mentioned old wives' tales- please don't just go and try any old theory that you hear, without doing proper research and speaking to a healthcare practitioner about it first.

And ice? Ice slows histamines. It doesn't stop them, but it gives you time to put BUTTER on! (Or something else that you find helps your bruises).

What also goes a long way is getting out of moves nicely. That's right, it's really all about posture, stabilising your positions, placing your limbs, and even dismounting the pole! If you release and plop out of moves, you'll put undue strain on your joints, especially your shoulders. Once you start to get a spin, practise landing it. Getting into the habit of landing nicely will mean that if you have a bad day, niceties will be all your body knows, and no one will notice. However, if you're having a bad day and your body is used to plonking out of moves, you're more likely to cause an

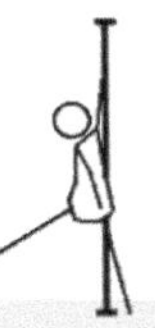

injury. Bad days are usually your body's way of telling you it's tired and needs a rest, so don't push it. Activate muscles, control, and land nicely every time.

On the topic of looking after your body, you don't want to look like a one-armed lobster with one shoulder rippling with muscles and one spaghetti arm. Train your left and your right. When you recap moves you know, start on your weaker side. You always spend more time training the side you start on, so mix it up. Training both sides is imperative to keeping your body safe, keeping everything aligned and balanced, and avoiding causing an injury. Plus, when you get to going upside down, you want to know that whichever hand you put down to get out of a tricky situation is strong.

I found that there were some moves I couldn't get on one side but could do on the other. Give up on a frustrating move and try the other side. Your muscle balance or flexibility may be different, and whammy, you've got it! Then go back to the first side, and your body will have a better idea of what it's doing.

Pole is amazing for strength and postural stability, but you need to work at a balanced rate within your personal limits. Otherwise, there is a risk of injury.[16]

Warm Up and Cool Down

Yep, I'm still rabbiting on about keeping yourself safe. It's an overwhelming amount of information, but having a well-rounded idea of what you are getting into early on makes the journey so much easier and safer.

The next things to consider are your warm-up and cool-down routines. Your body needs to know what's coming. It can't just wake up and do as you ask without feeling like sloppy lettuce afterwards. I do the same chest, arm, and shoulder stretches at the beginning and end of each training session, and I do these on the pole, as it helps the pole warm up too, which can sometimes help with grip; it also helps my squeal factor when putting a metal pole between my thighs!

Next, I consider what I'll be training and do some stretches to suit those moves specifically. I love creating warm-up routines to music, starting slow and moving through each part of my body. This helps me combat the old-school 'sit down and stretch' mentality.

One thing about static stretching is that it affects the length of your muscles. Okay. You stretched it. Wasn't that the aim? But this can reduce the ability of muscles to contract and produce muscle strength. There's no winning!

Dynamic stretching, however, can be a lot of fun. It more effectively goes through the full range of motion of each muscle group or area. It gets your blood pumping and your heart rate up and is proven to increase flexibility more than static stretching.

Passive stretching alone doesn't get your body warm and doesn't use the full range of motion of your muscles and joints, so it leaves you more prone to injury. Some more advanced split moves are quite passive on the pole, so there may be space for passive stretching there, but that's a while away!

I create warm-up routines that include body rolls, kicks, and hip, chest, wrist, elbow, and arm circles, covering each area of the body. Mix stretching with music, and get your blood pumping and your body warm. That way, you'll be ready to train safely!

You'll notice as you go through this book that I've included muscles to stretch and strengthen for each move. This is so that you can put together your training program, creating your dynamic warm-up and exercises to suit the moves you're working on.

Please be aware that you should always stretch within your comfort zone. Pushing too hard can cause injury. If choosing to incorporate static stretches in your routine, holding static stretches for 10 seconds is generally enough. Longer than 30 seconds gives no flexibility benefits.[6] Keep in mind your body's limitations; everyone's body is different and has different mobility restrictions and structures that may limit their flexibility. Whether it be muscle or nerve tension, joint mobility, or something else, your range of motion is different to someone else; work within your own limits to decrease the risk of injury.

Want to go into more detail? Don't stress! There's a warm-up section later in this book!

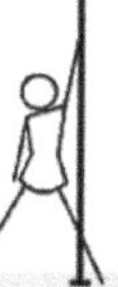

Warming Up on the Pole

I like turning my warm-ups into a dance. This way, I can raise my pulse and get my joints moving. Plus, it makes preparing to train fun instead of a chore. I also include a brief run-through of separate dynamic range-of-motion-based stretches to wake my shoulders and chest up, as well as any other specific moves.

Remember, dynamic warm-ups and stretching are proven to be more efficient than static stretches. It's amazing how easy it is to put on some music and just start moving, focusing on one body part at a time, moving from top to bottom or bottom to top.

Getting your arms moving with your neck works well as a combo, or watch the direction your hands go, warming up your arms and neck at the same time. If you bring one arm out to the side and up in a semicircle, doing a hip push to that same side, watch your hand come up and down, pushing your hip to the other side. Then swap sides.

Hip circles, chest circles, and body rolls are also fantastic warm-ups. High kicks and side kicks are amazing. Just check when kicking that your movement is coming from your leg, not your torso. Keep your torso upright as you kick, and be aware of where the pole is in your space.

I like doing squat steps, squatting down and coming up to tap the foot to one side, then going back to a squat and tapping to the other side. Remember your alignment. Make sure that your knee never goes over your toes in a squat, or you may cause injury.

Play around with leg/knee/foot isolations. How can you move them to music smoothly and repetitively? Rotate your knee up, then to the side and down, or lift your leg, keeping your knee still, and mix with your foot, creating little isolated circles. Can you squat down and pivot to one side, then back to the other? Can you do slow half neck rolls that work with the music?

You could even start in one spot, say your wrist or hand. Start movement, just circles, then allow that movement to grow. Let it get bigger and bigger, then move to the elbow, then to the shoulder, then the torso. Then add the neck and legs. You could recreate an oceanic rumbling water scenario, adding one extra part of your body at a time.

With kids, I tell stories about the weather, and we recreate what we think it would be like to be in a tornado or what heavy rain looks like. We even do natural disasters and volcanoes! They love hanging themselves on the 'clothesline' to dry and flapping their limbs in the wind or flying through space to different planets as we dodge comets. What about recreating ocean creatures? What would your octopus look like? Don't feel limited to the conventional. Picking a scenario or an animal and working out matching movements is a fun warm-up, and it allows you to move in different ways than you would normally.

Warm-ups don't have to be boring, so have some fun. As long as you're moving each part of your body in a safe manner and not going too intense with it, that's what you're aiming for here. Make the movement yours! Use it to help you find your flow of the day. What music are you feeling? Move to that, one joint at a time, and lose yourself in the music.

I get it. Sometimes, you just want someone to tell you what to do and not be given options to figure out yourself. Here are a few of my staple warm-up moves.

Kicks

Standing side on to the pole, holding the pole with your inside hand, keeping your torso upright and hips and shoulders square, kick your outside leg forward and back. Then swap to the other side. Want an aim? Find a visual spot, and try to reach it. I like to aim to kick my light as a visual height cue.

When aiming to push higher, make sure you keep your shoulders and torso upright and that you're not crouching over to gain momentum. The movement is from the hips. Only go as far as you feel comfortable. Don't throw it and do a hammy (tear a hamstring muscle, for non-Aussies!).

I then turn to face the pole, holding on with both hands. I swing one leg between me and the pole and out to the side. Again, watch your posture here. Keep your shoulders up and your body square and aligned. Be careful not to kick the pole. I find the most likely time to kick the pole is when you're about to move on and are less focused on that leg. Do both sides.

Arm circles

If you don't want to do choreographed arm and neck rolls, you can do big arm circles forward and backward. You can even swing and wrap them from side to side like you're in a washing machine.

Neck rolls

Neck rolls are a funny one. Everyone has something different to say. I heard a long time ago that full neck rolls aren't good for you, and it stuck in my mind, so I do semicircles, ear to shoulder, around the front and to the other shoulder and back.

I feel uncomfortable taking my neck back anyway, so this suits me fine. Depending on what you're doing, you can add extra stretches in, but remember not to put pressure on your neck; it's delicate!

Squat kicks

Holding on to the pole with 2 hands, squat back and down. Remember, in a squat, your knees should be above your ankles, and your legs should be at 90 degrees with your thighs parallel to the floor so that your hips and knees are aligned. The pole helps with this alignment.

Stand up out of the squat, and bend one leg behind you as if you're going to kick your bottom. Squat, stand up, kick your other foot to your bottom, and repeat. Depending on the music I'm using, I like going into a squat and raising onto the balls of my feet, one at a time, then coming to stand and lowering back to flat feet. If you have a good beat, you can do it to the music.

Chest circles, hip circles, and body rolls

I always include some chest circles, hip circles. and body rolls. They really get you moving! There are a few options for you to play with. Just make sure you move through every joint and get your blood flowing. Still need more structure? Have a look at the next couple of pages for some ideas.

Warming Up: Working Down Your Body

(example only)

- Finger flicks.
- Finger spreads (wide, then together, wide, then together)
- Talking hand puppets
- Wrist shakes
- Wrist circles
- Waves with arms (interlocked fingers)

- Bring ear to one shoulder. Rotate neck forward, then circle other ear to shoulder.
- Look up to the sky and down to the floor.
- Look over right and left shoulders.

- Chest slides (left, right, forward, back)
- Chest openers (forward and back, pulling arms with you, opposite way to the chest)
- Chest circles

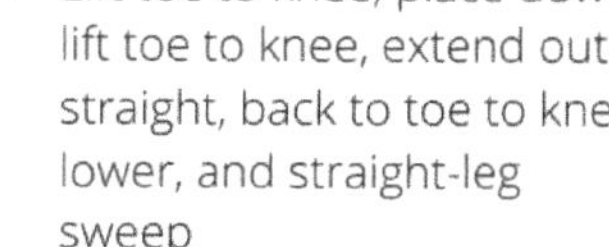

- Shoulder rolls
- Elbow circles (both directions)
- Arm circles (forward, backward, then one forward and one backward)
- Arm swings (up and down, swapping directions)
- ·Hold hands together, circle arms over head, behind you, around head, and to front
- Washing machine arm wraps (soft knees), twisting body to side and letting arms flow and wrap around you, then back again
- ·Step out to the side and reach or punch across body with opposite arm
- Side lean, opposite arm reaching up and over head, rotate to flat back, circle down leg to flat back on other side

- High-knee walk/jog
- Kicking bottom run
- Hips side to side (can add straight-arm pulses)
- Hip circles
- Hip openers (knee up and around to the outside and down)
- Lift toe to knee, place down, lift toe to knee, extend out straight, back to toe to knee, lower, and straight-leg sweep
- High kicks (keep torso upright)
- Lunge back, then stand to kick (holding pole)
- Side kicks (across front, then out to side)
- Jump with hip twist
- Forward bend (reach forward, middle, and through the legs; then reach each leg with opposite arm)
- Side lunge (rotate from one side to the other)
- Lift knee to 90 degrees, keep stationary, and draw circle with foot
- Squat down, come up, and point one foot to side

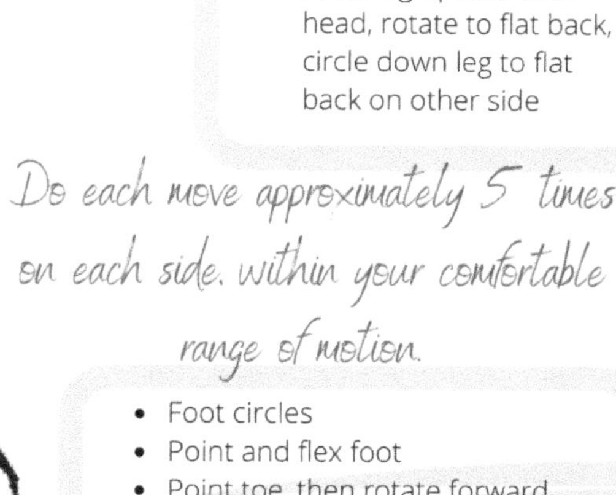

Do each move approximately 5 times on each side. within your comfortable range of motion.

- Foot circles
- Point and flex foot
- Point toe, then rotate forward over toes, back to point, and down

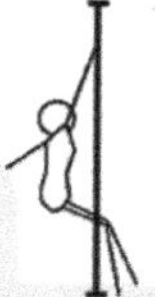

Warm-up options need to include 3 to 5 minutes of cardio, including hip, neck, wrist, and shoulder rotations. Here are some cardio ideas for you to consider. For most moves, consider doing 5 moves on each side, and have some fun playing with arm and leg combinations. Start with the more natural movements (walking, jogging), increasing the range of motion to create bigger movements. Then work to smaller, more intricate movements. Remember; your hands hold you up, they need some care and to be warmed up too!

Ensure that you also focus on movements that directly relate to what you're training. For example, I always do some ground movements that are similar before moving to windmills on the floor, then windmills up the pole.

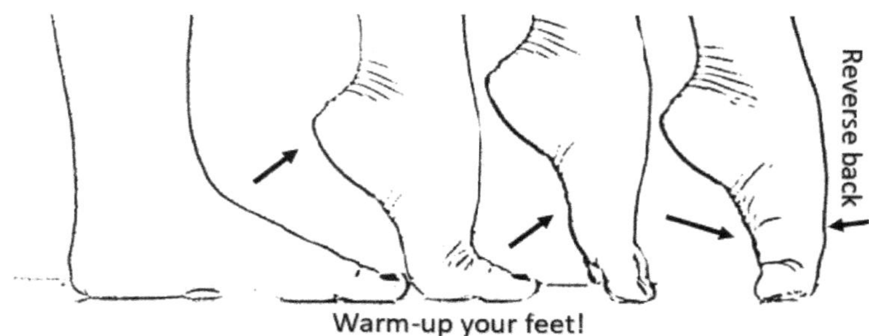

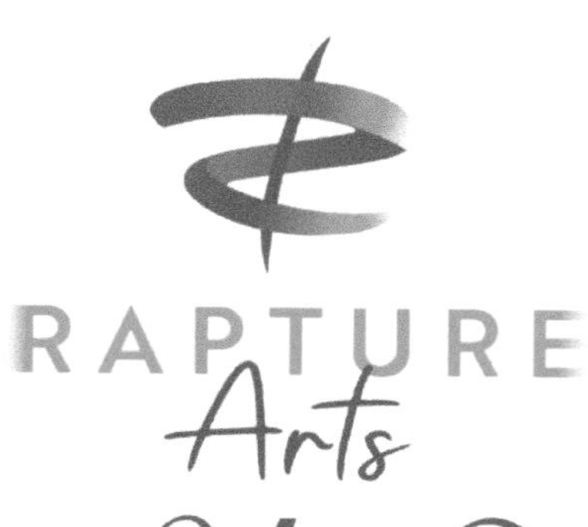

Warm Up Options

MOVE	REPS	THINGS TO THINK OF
Inhale as arms come up; exhale while circling them down	2 or 3 depending on your tension	Focus on breathing. This is a calming way to start and finish.
Punching (straight, uppercut, and side hook)	5 sets of each on each side	Practise safe habits, even for fitness. Never tuck your thumbs in to punch.
Jog forward and backward (optional finger flicks or punches)		Always look where you're going! If jogging is too intense, try a brisk walk
Kick-bottom run	x10	I like to squat down and push/step up to kick bottom instead of running.
High-knee run	x10	High-knee walk if a run is too intense.
Star jumps (jumping jacks)	2 on each side	Add in jump quarter-turns so that you can do a whole circle
Side step (arms going out and in optional)	5 to the left; 5 to the right	To add more cardio, do a little jump in the air as your feet come together.
Grapevine	5 to the left; 5 to the right	Combine up and down arm movements to make a full-body exercise.
Skipping	20 seconds	Play with variations with or without skipping rope. (beware of surroundings)
Rowing	30 seconds	This is an amazing exercise for pole!
High Kicks (can also do side kicks)	5 left; 5 right	Keep your torso straight and upright. Think of a string holding you up tall.
Crab walk	5 left; 5 right	If too strenuous, pick another animal- e.g. frog?
Lunge walks	5 left; 5 right	Ensure your ankle and knee are aligned. You don't want your front knee going over your toes.
Arm, elbow and wrist circles	5 forwards; 5 backwards	

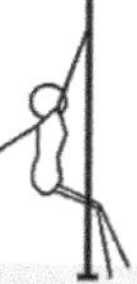

Always listen to your body and work within your limitations. Maintaining safe alignment.

Working with Gravity: First Moves

Now you have strong background knowledge, know where you're at, have stretched, and are warm and ready to start. But where?

Let's just double-check. You are stretched and warm, right? That's super important injury protection. Please don't forget it. Make a routine of it every training session.

Let me take you through some moves. I've found that these slowly build onto the next moves, creating a stable foundation for your future training.

I've also included some of the main muscles or areas used in each skill and what you may want to work on with strengthening or stretching. I want you to be aware that there are other stabilising muscles also involved. The muscles I list are only listed as a base guide to give you an idea of what your body is doing and to help you work out what you may need to activate, strengthen, or stretch.

My recommendation is to start with the **basic fireman spin**. I say this for several reasons. Using the **basic spin grip**, you can start to get comfortable with your arm strength before progressing to more complicated grips. This grip protects your joints when learning. This spin also has the most skin contact on the pole, offering better grip so that your arms aren't taking all the strain initially. In this move, you can literally hold on for dear life and realise that you have the strength to hold you there! It's also very similar to the foetal position, making it your safest-feeling position primally as well. It's a good foundation, and having an understanding of it leads you on to so many more things.

Now, when you start pole, one of the things to get accustomed to is that we don't use left and rights, as we train both sides, and as you progress, there can be lots to think of, without worrying about your left or right side. Instead, we talk about inside and outside. Inside being the closest limb to the pole, Outside is the farthest away arm or leg to the pole. This way, it doesn't matter what side of the pole you stand or which way around you are; it is easier to orientate yourself.

Basic Spin Grip

Let's start by taking a look at your grip. This is the **basic spin grip (also known as thumb-up grip)**.

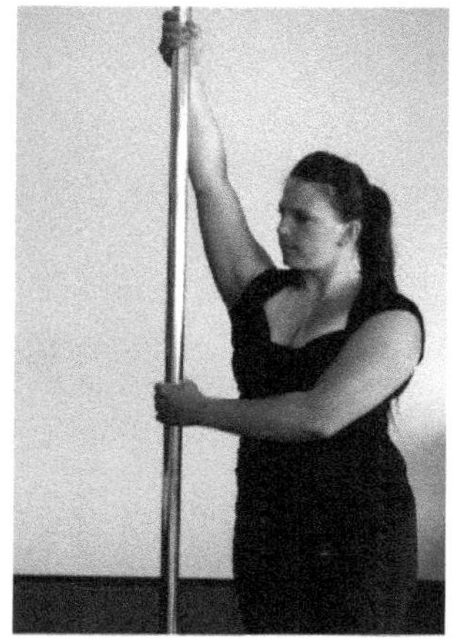

Place your inside hand up high. Keep your elbow straight; if you don't, you'll feel like you need to lift with your bicep. Your palm should face the direction you're going in. Now roll your shoulders back and down to activate them. This encourages you to lift more with your shoulders. You'll actively pull with this arm as you spin.

Bring your outside hand across your body, and hold on at chest or waist height. Waist height generally allows for more of a push with the bottom arm so that your pelvis doesn't come towards the pole. When gripping, you should always think of a push/pull scenario (pull with the top; push with the bottom). This hand placement can vary depending on your body's proportions.

Bam! That's your first grip! Meet your **basic spin grip**.

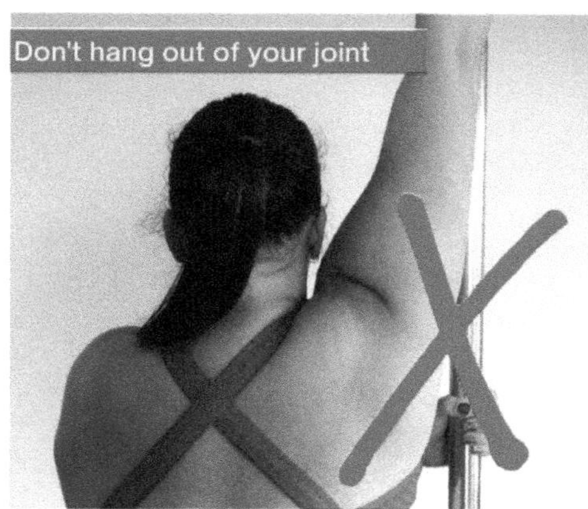

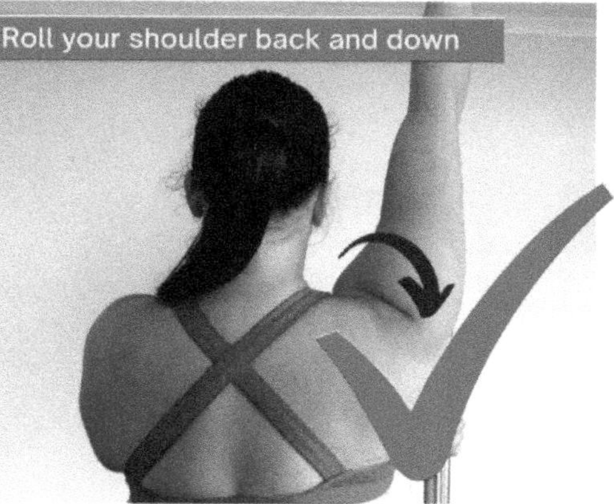

If you struggle to get your outside hand across your front, you may want to consider more of a baseball grip, having the bottom hand up higher on the pole, leaving a gap from your top hand as if you were holding a baseball bat. Another alternative is to tuck your bottom hand below your breasts (for females). This is high enough to still create a straight line through your wrist to the pole without extending the grip too low to put excess pressure on your wrist by creating a bend in it. You may find that this is your preferred option if you have more tender wrists.

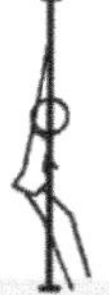

As mentioned, generally, grips focus on a push/pull scenario. Your top arm in this situation is your 'spinning arm'. Your outside arm works to help support your weight and steer your body.

Muscles/Areas to Strengthen for the Basic Spin Grip

- Shoulder girdle and scapular stabilisers (trapezius, serratus anterior)
- Rotator cuff (teres minor, infraspinatus)
- Pectorals

Muscles to Stretch for the Basic Spin Grip

- Triceps
- Latissimus dorsi
- Pectorals

BASIC SPIN GRIP

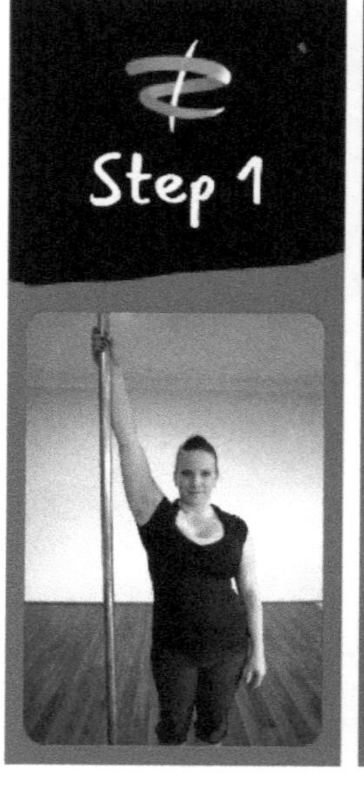

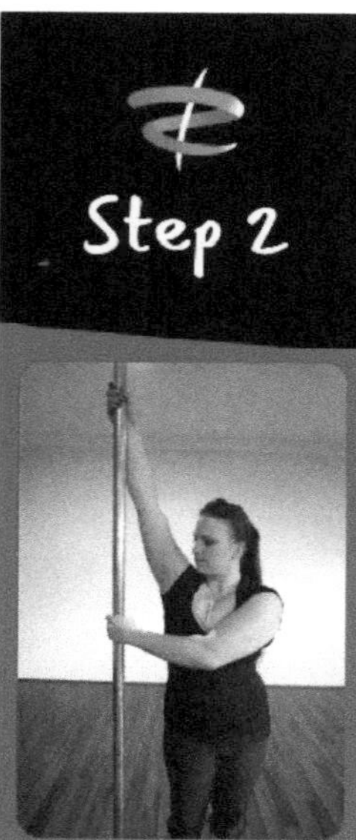

<u>Remember:</u>

- Your top palm always faces the direction that you are going.
- Roll your shoulders back and down.

Now to focus on the rest of the body! Deadlifting into moves this early on sucks! Use momentum and velocity to help hold you up. Basically, walk into your spins; don't just lift into them. Some lift is required so that you don't hang off of your shoulder joint. That's why we roll our shoulders back initially, but if you think of lifting, you tend to bend your top elbow, and that makes you use a whole new set of muscles and is actually harder. It's best not to think of the lift! I think of flowing my body in the direction of the momentum, so, if you are walking forwards, think of maintaining that forwards motion as you spin, instead of thinking about taking your feet off the ground, as that makes you more likely to lift than flow forwards.

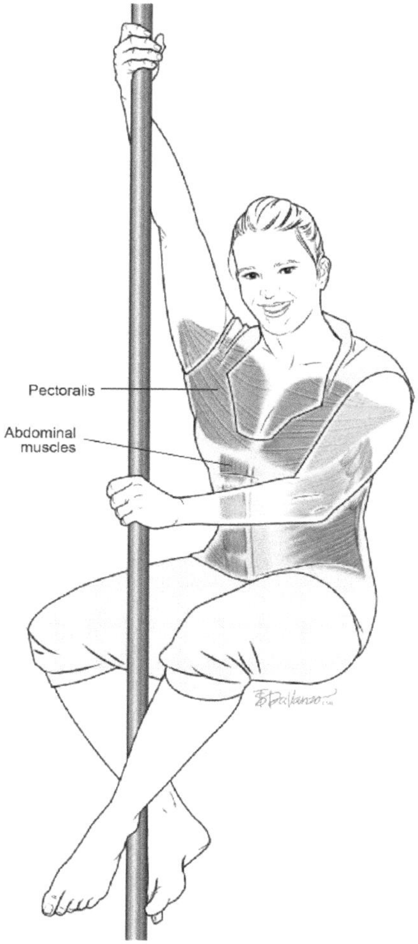

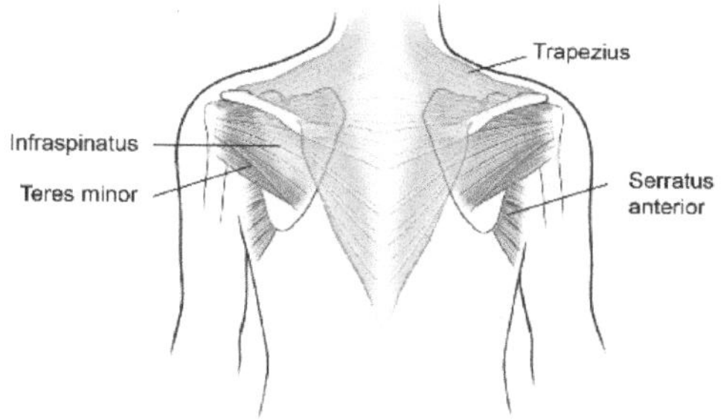

The Basic Fireman Spin

Start with your hands in the **basic spin grip**. What you're going to do next is take a step on your inside leg. This frees you up to bring your outside leg around the front of the pole so that your knee is on one side and your foot is on the other, slightly diagonal. You should have all of the skin of your calf on the pole and your knee at around hip height, no higher. The other leg will tap behind the pole, knee on one side,

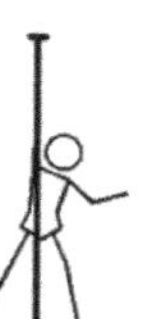

foot on the other. Again, all skin should touch the pole. Welcome to your **basic fireman position**. Now practise it with a walk to give you a bit of momentum to help the spin. I find three steps is a good count; you can start on the step/foot that you want to start your spin on, one, two, three, on three, you are back on that spinning foot and can go straight into the spin.

Let's take a look.

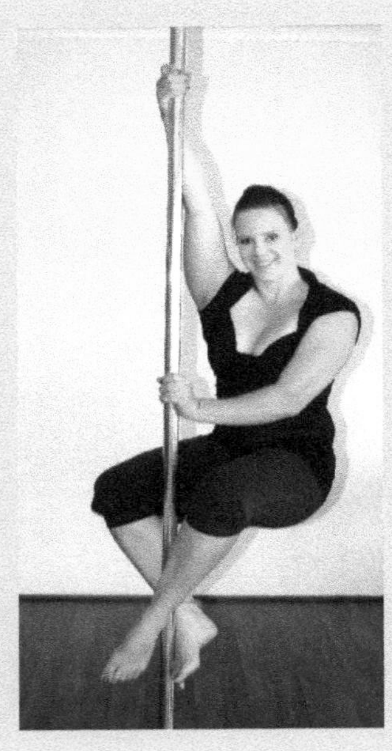

Step 1: Place your inside hand up, palm facing the direction you're going in, and roll your shoulder back.

Step 2: Put your outside hand across your body, holding on at waist height.

Step 3: Step on your inside leg to bring your outside leg in front of the pole (knee on one side, ankle on the other).

Step 4: Tap your other leg to the back of the pole (knee on one side, ankle on the other so that one knee is on each side of the pole).

Step 5: Spin!

Muscles/Areas to Strengthen for the Fireman

- Hip flexors
- Shoulder girdle and scapular stabilisers (trapezius, serratus anterior)
- Rotator cuff (teres minor, infraspinatus)
- Core (abs, back, and pelvic floor)

Muscles to Stretch for the Fireman

- Glutes
- Hamstrings
- Triceps
- Latissimus dorsi
- Pectorals

Please be aware that every pole move has a high focus on all core muscles – abdominals and spinal muscle groups. The pelvic floor is one of those forgotten muscles, but if activated, it assists with alignment so much! Even if these muscles

VISUALISATION: BASIC FIREMAN

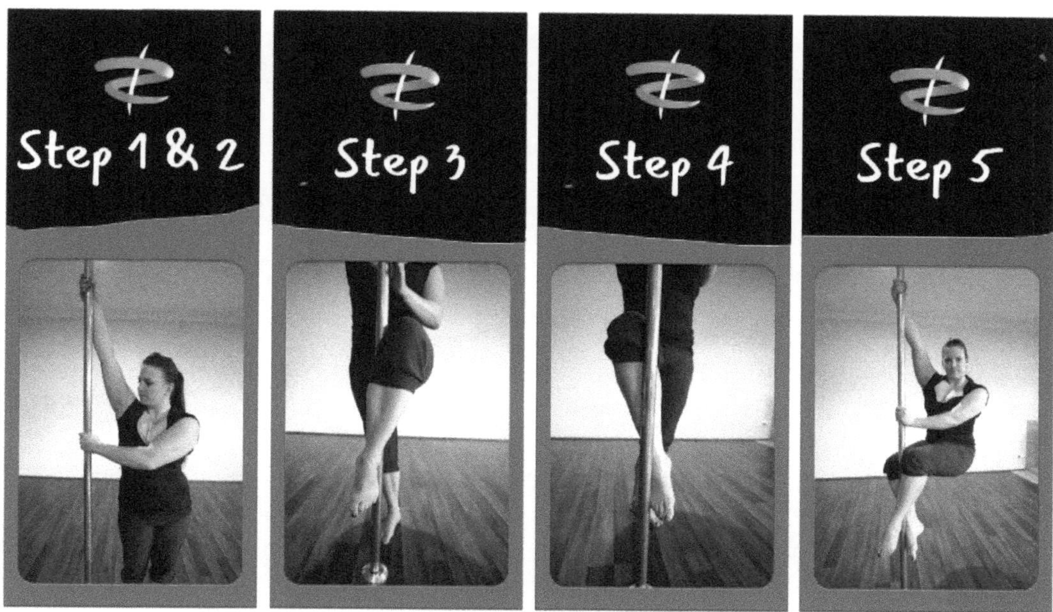

You would be keeping your front leg on the pole for step 4; the image is just showing leg placement.

aren't listed as groups to strengthen with each move, they are muscles to always consider in your conditioning regime.

Don't forget to try this move on both sides. Think of each step one at a time. The other side might feel odd initially. Just remember: inside hand, then outside hand (not left, then right!). Having a solid metal object in your space is not normal, and it will take some getting used to, so don't stress. Just practise away! Momentum does really help hold you in the spin, so once you are comfortable with your position it is really satisfying to play with the momentum in, and smoothly coming out of the move too.

Now, I know the words won't help everyone, but they are great cues once you know how to move around the pole a bit. To help that solidify and make sense, scan the QR code, which will take you to a video to help you piece it together.

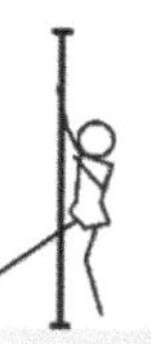

Got that! What's next? The next 2 are a bit funny. The move after this is easier than this one, but it's best to do this next one first. If it's not clicking for you, that's fine. Move on to the next move, then come back, and you may find it all falls into place for you.

The Front Knee Hook Spin

Now for your front-knee hook (also known as forward-knees) spin. Again, you'll need to use your **basic spin grip**, so place your arms, roll your shoulders back, and focus on your legs. Ready?

Pick up your inside leg, and bring it around the front of the pole, bending at the knee. Do this at a comfortable height, not too high. Then go up onto your tippy-toes with your outside leg. This realigns your hips. Now think of falling forward, leaning through your hips, bending your other leg as you go. My 6-year-old calls it 'Santa belly' (sticking your belly out to make it as big as possible).

The trick to this one is all in the hips. If there's a bend in your torso/hips, you'll feel as if your arms are taking much more weight and your muscles are working hard. Once everything is aligned with the hips forward, it's so much easier. This spin uses gravity to do the work. Take this down to the ground.

Why take it down to the ground? By going down to the ground, you are holding the move longer, so at this point, it is two extra seconds of conditioning that you would not have otherwise had. This conditioning all builds up; but going to the ground also lets you focus on the move, rather than the dismount.

You can also play with fun poses or lean backs after you land and practise getting up. Eventually, you can practise getting out of this move without going to the ground, but for now, the extra conditioning time helps. Don't worry about where the pole sits on your leg. This will differ from person to person depending on differences in bodies and builds.

Are you ready?

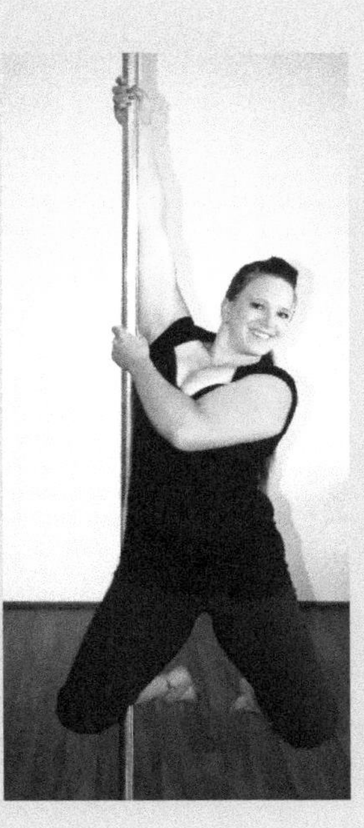

Step 1: Place your inside hand up, palm facing the direction you're going in, and roll your shoulder back.

Step 2: Place your outside hand across your body, holding on at waist height.

Step 3: Bend your inside leg onto the pole.

Step 4: Stand up on your tippy-toes on your outside leg.

Step 5: Lean forward through your hips, bending your other leg when you need to. Let gravity do the work!

Step 6: Spin to the floor! Again and again, then on the other side too.

There are 2 variations for legs: feet apart and in line with your knee or diamond toes pointing to each other. Some people find creating a diamond with their feet helps get their hips forward; others don't. If you're struggling, it's worth giving a shot!

VISUALISATION: FRONT KNEE-HOOK

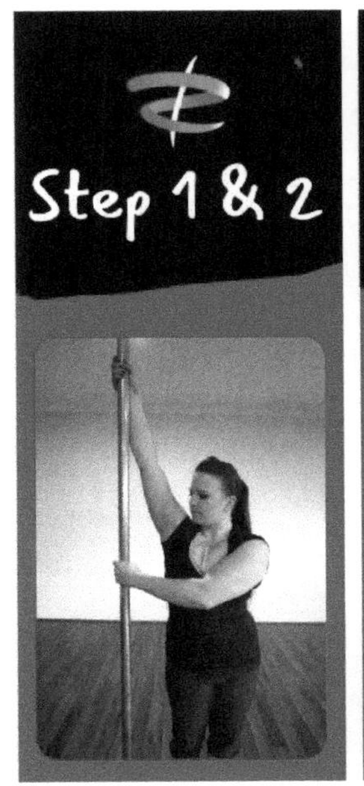

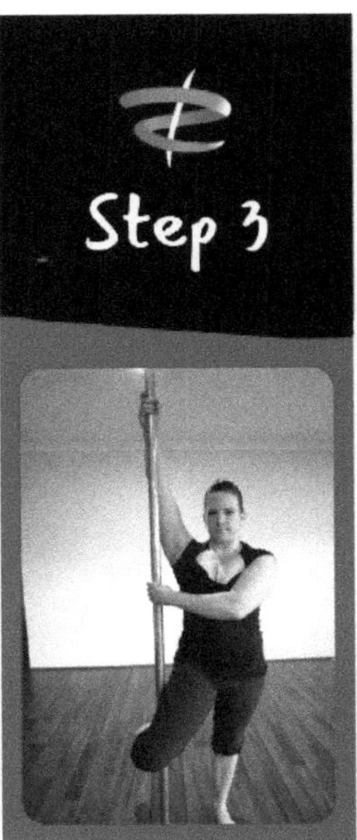

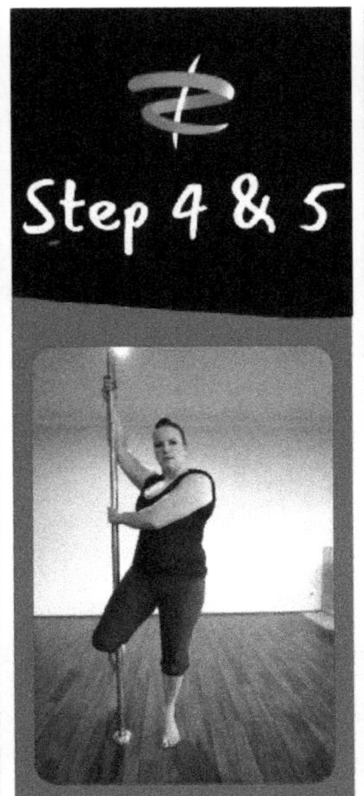

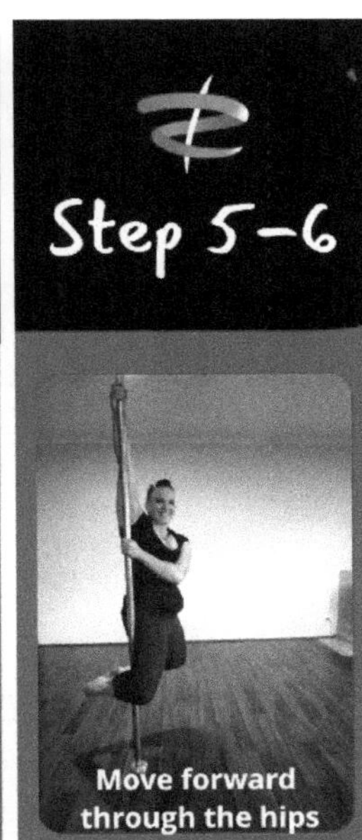

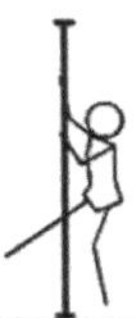

Muscles/Areas to Strengthen for the Front-Knee Hook

- Shoulder girdle and scapular stabilisers (trapezius, serratus anterior)
- Rotator cuff (teres minor, infraspinatus)
- Pectorals
- Hamstrings
- Core (including pelvic floor)

Muscles to Stretch for the Front-Knee Hook

- Hip flexors
- Quads
- Triceps
- Latissimus dorsi

Like I said, the next one is actually easier. That's because your body is already in the right position. Your hips are already forward. The hardest thing is convincing your head that it's okay to go backward, which is why we didn't do this move first.

Reverse Spin Grip

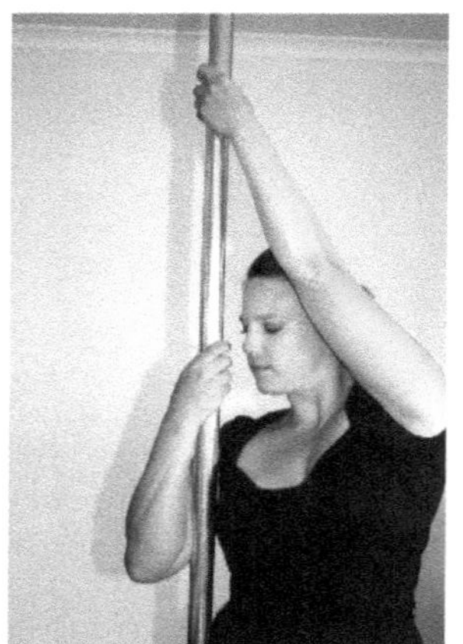

This means you need to learn your **reverse spin grip**! When you go backward, your outside hand is on top, and your palm always faces the direction you're going.

I have a habit of applying a bit of force when I grab the pole to go back. This way, if it's like you're hitting the pole (lightly, of course) and your hand is the wrong way around, it will be more obvious, as you won't feel stable, whereas if your hand is facing the right way, it will feel like you've just got a solid grasp. Moral of the story: palm faces the direction you intend to go! That's your outside hand. Your inside hand wraps in next to you at shoulder height. Don't forget to roll your shoulder back before setting your grip. This is your **reverse spin grip**.

Muscles/Areas to Strengthen for the Reverse Spin Grip

- Shoulder girdle and scapular stabilisers (trapezius, serratus anterior)
- Rotator cuff (teres minor, infraspinatus)

Muscles to Stretch for the Reverse Spin Grip

- Triceps
- Latissimus dorsi
- Quadratus lumborum (side or lateral trunk flexors)
- Pectorals

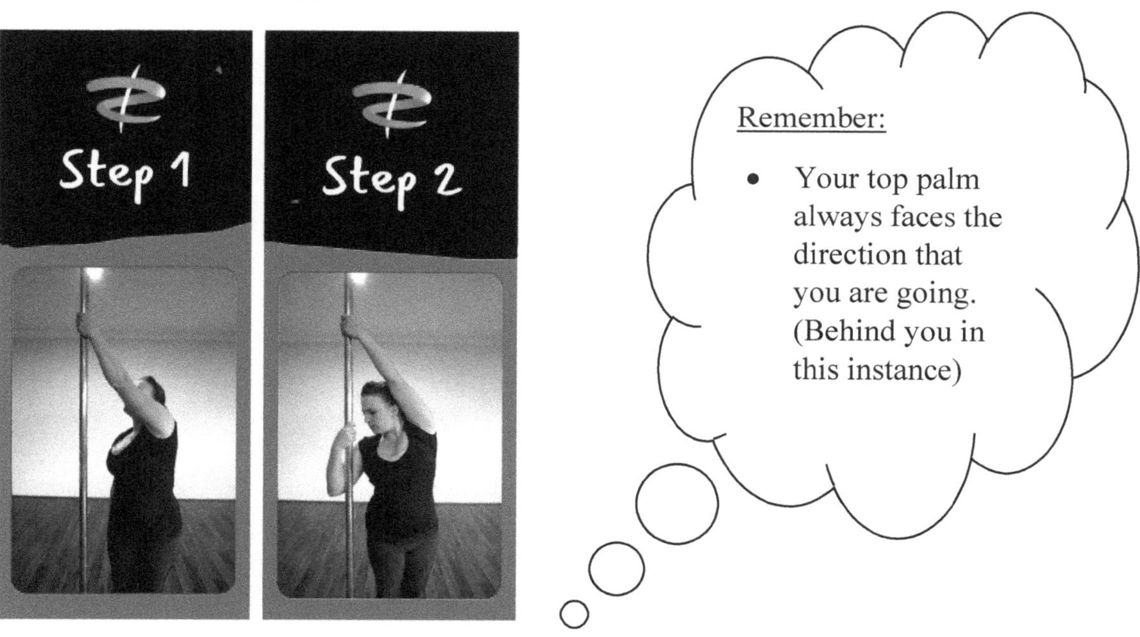

The Back-knee hook

Now for the back-knee hook (also known as backward-knees) spin!

Set yourself, with your shoulders rolled back, side on to the pole in your **reverse spin grip**. Now it's time for the legs. Take your inside leg in front of the pole on its toe. If you give your heel a bit of a wiggle, it shouldn't hit the pole. If your foot is too far away, you won't feel stable (you'll feel like you're falling), so keep it reasonably close.

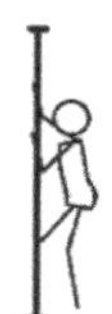

Now transfer weight onto the ball of that foot. Bring your outside leg out in front of you, then around to the side and behind you, like you're using your toe to draw a circle around yourself and the pole. Let your body move with this motion, rotating on the ball of your foot. Once you feel comfortable with this move, you can really push all of your body weight down your outside leg to the toe as your draw your circle. This creates a straight line from your top, outside hand to your outside toe. This straight-line really helps you feel stronger as well as more safe and secure in entering this move, as well as gaining you momentum for the spin.

As your leg comes behind you, bend it. When the inside of your calf touches the pole, bend your leg around the pole and spin to the floor. If you try and jump into this or bend your leg before your calf touches, you're asking for a bruise! Spin this one down to the floor as well. You can work on transitions to standing later.

Let's do it.

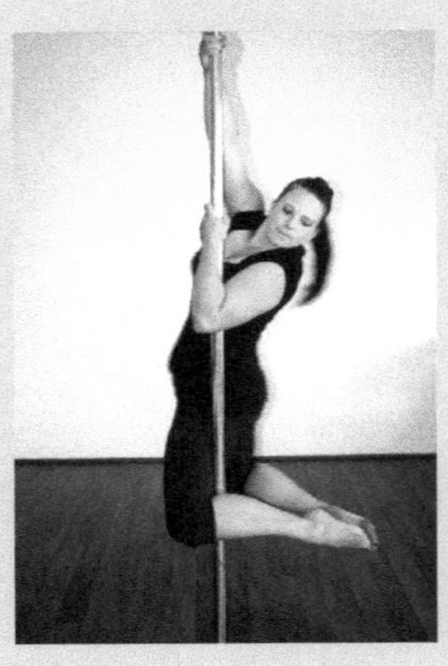

Step 1: Roll your shoulder back. Put your outside hand up, palm facing the direction you're going (behind you).

Step 2: Wrap your inside hand around the pole at shoulder height.

Step 3: Place your inside foot on its toe in front of the pole. Give it a wiggle to make sure you don't hit the pole.

Step 4: Transfer your weight onto the ball of your inside foot.

Step 5: Use the toe of your outside leg to draw a circle around you, starting in front and going behind you.

Step 6: As your calf touches the pole, bend your knees.

Step 7: Spin down to the ground. Again and again, then practise the other side too.

You have another new grip and direction to play with in this move. Have a look at the QR code to help you piece it together. Another video awaits!

BACK KNEE HOOK

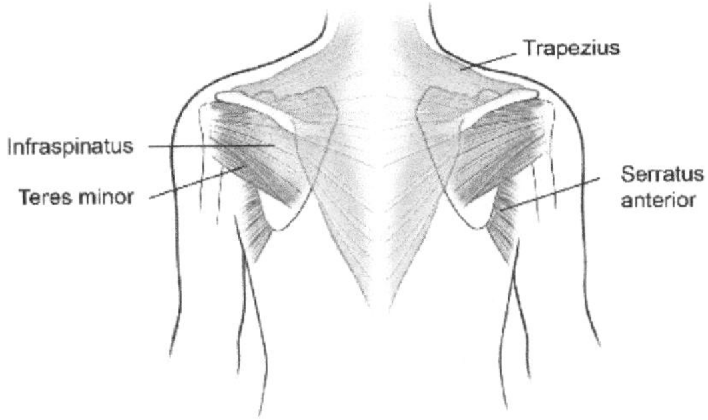

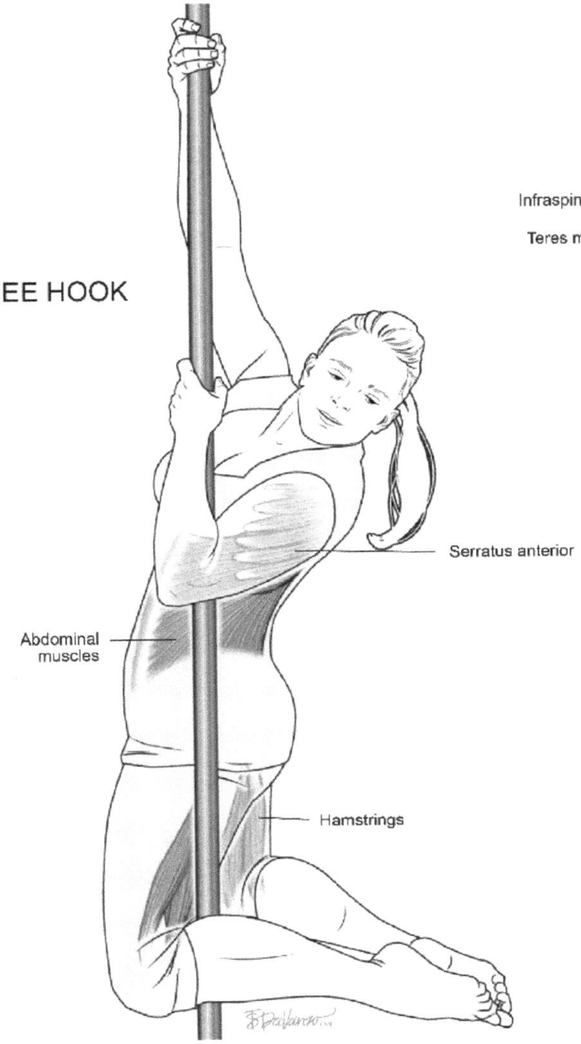

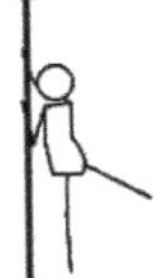

VISUALISATION: BACK KNEE-HOOK

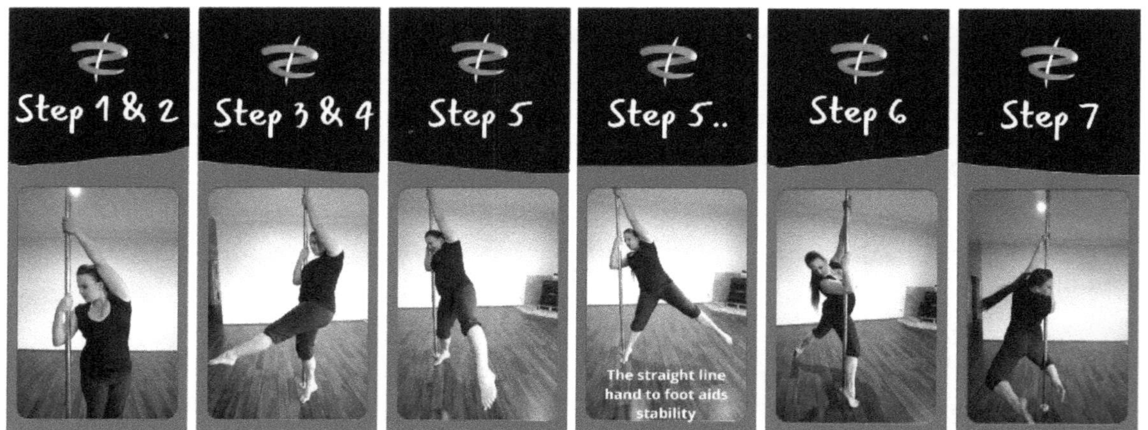

Muscles/Areas to Strengthen for the Back-Knee Hook

- Shoulder girdle and scapular stabilisers (trapezius, serratus anterior)
- Rotator cuff (teres minor, infraspinatus)
- Hamstrings
- Core muscles (including pelvic floor)

Muscles to Stretch for the Back-Knee Hook

- Hip flexors
- Quads
- Triceps
- Latissimus dorsi
- Quadratus lumborum (side or lateral trunk flexors)

Other good things to practise at this stage are pole walks, bows, poses, hip circles, body rolls, and pivots and pirouettes on one foot to bring you back to the pole.

In every session, look at starting training for lifts, using your arms, just above head height, to lift you onto your tippy-toes. If that's too easy, lift your feet off the ground. If you find that you're inclined to jump, try kneeling. That way, you can't push off your feet to lift, though you will have to lift your whole body up, not just lifting to your toes! Gradual baby steps and starting early make it easier to lift later.

Ensure that you practice moves that you have previously been working on each training session. Each move has so many little parts to it. Lots of steps and elements, not just physically but mentally. I find that you focus so much on one part of a move that it finally clicks, and then you find there is another part to work on next! Eventually, it gets there, but also, I have noticed that, after a training session, working on a particular thing, once I have finished, it is like all the little neural pathways in your brain link it together. When you come back, things seem to click a bit more. Take it one step at a time, don't rush the journey and you will get there!

There is a couple of spins to practice, but one of the strange things about pole, is one of the simplest of things. Moving and flowing around it, basic walking! It sounds silly, but have you tried flat footed walking around a pole?! It just doesn't cut it!

Walking around a pole can feel very alien. Having a solid metal object in your space can feel totally strange, then to walk around it?! If you walk normally, you just get dizzy! I find if I walk, crossing one foot over the other with each step, it almost tricks your body into walking in a circle, with out even realising it. This allows for you to not get so dizzy, but also gives the awesome curve effect of your hips as you walk. You can do these as little steps, with big exaggerated kick backs before stepping, even little Latino style twists as you walk, twist it up and down, play with the music, what flows with the beat? Always ensure your outside hand has a job, your inside hand is holding the pole, every now and then you will pop onto the balls of your feet and slide your inside hand up higher, you may find you pull with the top had, that is fine… but your outside hand can detract from everything. What is your floating hand in no-mans-land doing? Give it a purpose! Place it on your hip, run it through your hair, or down your side, cheekily point at someone- it is totally up to you, as long as it has a job and isn't making someone wonder what that hand is doing.

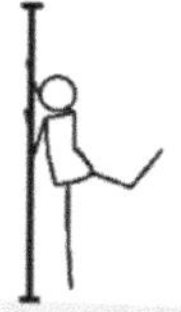

Stabilising Yourself and Your Grip

The moves you've done so far have hopefully started to click! It's time to change it up and add a new grip. We're going to introduce **split grip (also known as full-bracket or thumb-down grip)**.

By now, you know your arms can hold you, so you want to stabilise your body, not drop down into spins. Learning **split grip** early and getting used to it in your spins helps to stabilise your wrists and shoulders and makes life much easier with many more advanced moves. Learning now helps to correct little things and create alignment. It also opens up new options for spins.

If you're ever worried about going crotch-first into the pole, **split grip** is the perfect grip for this situation. It holds your body away from the pole, thus protecting your crotch!

Forearm Grip

If this grip is a bit much for you, think of pushing with your bottom hand in your **basic spin grip**. Also, start looking at exercises to help you develop your ability to lift your body weight with your arms. You can also have a play with a **forearm grip** to help build your push strength with your bottom arm. **Forearm grip** is a great stepping stone to help you understand how the push/pull technique with your hands works.

Practise from standing on the balls of your feet. While on your tippy-toes, lift one leg off the ground, pull with your top arm, and push with your bottom forearm (with your shoulders rolled back and activated). Try to lift your second leg off the floor. This will give you an idea of the grip and how the push/pull technique works. **Forearm grip** also allows you to practise the majority of **split grip** moves without putting strain on your bottom arm's forearm or wrist.

So, what are the steps for **forearm grip**?

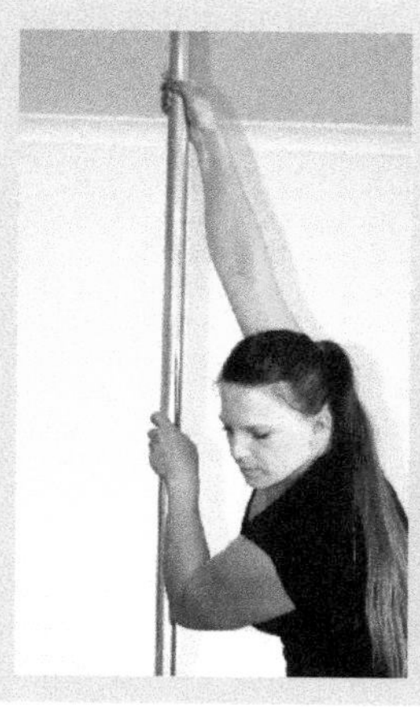

Step 1: Roll your shoulders back.

Step 2: Bring your inside hand up on the pole, arm straight, palm facing the direction you're going.

Step 3: Bring your outside hand in front of your face. (Like a little T-Rex arm.) Hold on to the pole, your forearm making contact down the pole.

Step 4: Pull with your top arm, and push with your bottom forearm. Voila: the **forearm grip**!

Split Grip

Next, you can look at trying **split grip kneeling**. Can you lift and slide your feet up to a squat? This makes more sense when you actually try it. You can also activate your **split grip** standing, lifting your legs slightly off the floor as you pull through the backs of your shoulders. This exercise is quite intense for the core muscles in the beginning.

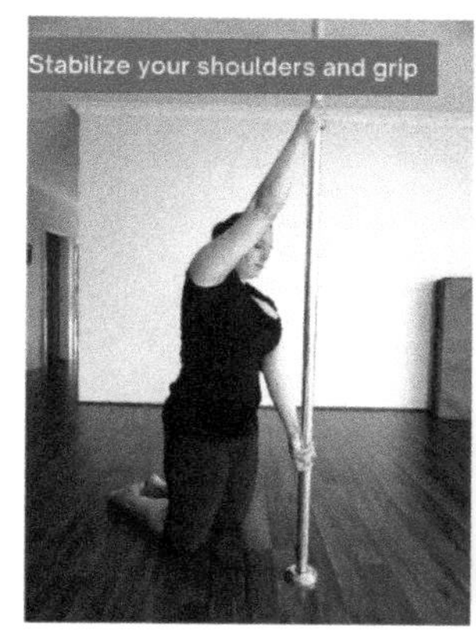

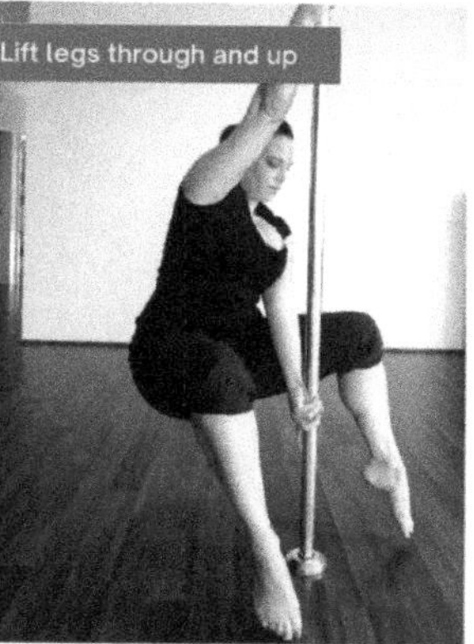

Right. Let's get on with it. How do you do the **split grip**?

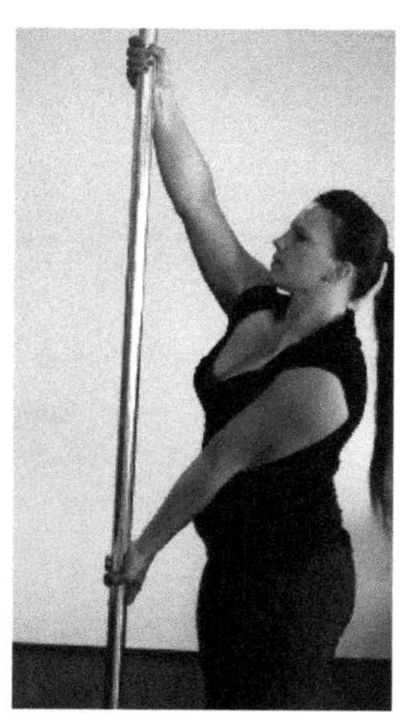

Roll your shoulders back, and place your inside hand high up on the pole. This is your pulling arm, and it needs to actively pull, not bend! Pull all the way into your shoulder blade. Place your outside hand low on the pole, pointer finger facing down, and push. If you have a look at the centre of the base of your palm, there's a valley in your hand, a little dip. Line this up with the centre of the pole. This helps to ensure that the bottom hand is coming straight onto the pole. This alone can lift you off the ground, but deadlifting into it sucks; the momentum of the spin helps dramatically!

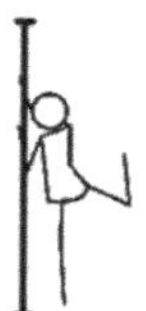

Now for the technical bits. If your finger isn't pointing down the pole, it changes your alignment. You want all the pressure going down your arm into the pole.

If that finger is wrapped, you'll notice that it pushes pressure past the pole and puts it all on the little bones and muscles in your wrists, straining them. You want your fingers to be relaxed here. Think of pushing the pole into the ground, like you're planting it.

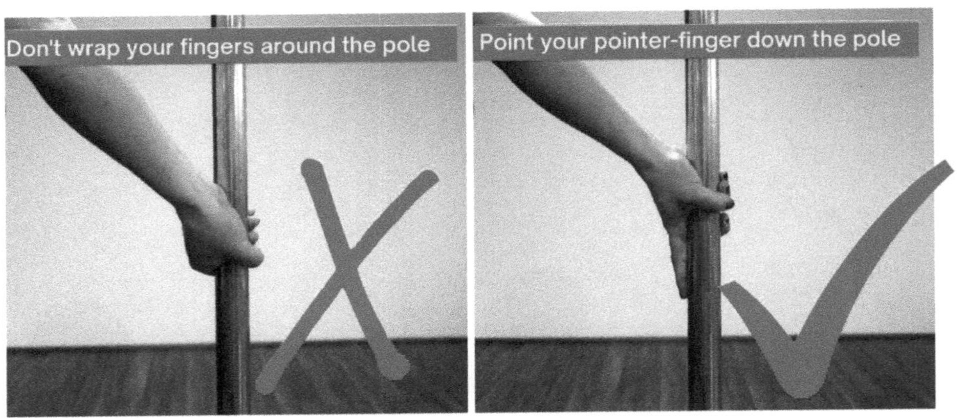

Next, look at your elbow. Does it hyperextend? You want the crease of your elbow to face the pole so that you're not locking your joints out. If you do have hyperextending elbows, you can practise going onto your hands and knees, setting your elbows straight. Then transfer weight into a plank/push-up position, focusing on holding your elbows in a neutral position. This helps strengthen them.

If you have incorrect alignment in this grip, you will get an ache in your forearm. This often comes from not pulling enough with your top arm (you don't want to hang in the joint). Self-check. Is everything straight? Are you actively pulling as well as pushing? Is your torso aligned, or are you throwing it out?

Walking into this grip can feel restricting and odd. This is how I get into it smoothly. This method also allows you to focus on setting one thing at a time.

Step 1: Roll your shoulders back. Place your inside hand up, palm facing the direction you're going.

Step 2: Step on your inside leg. Pivot to face the pole.

Step 3: Place your outside hand on the pole with your finger pointing down the pole.

*Please don't overdo this grip. Listen to your body. Doing too many grips in one session can cause strain and injury.

Muscles/Areas to Strengthen for the Split Grip

- Shoulder girdle and scapular stabilisers (trapezius, serratus anterior)
- Rotator cuff (teres minor, infraspinatus)
- Forearm flexors
- Elbow stability muscles (if hyper-extensive in the elbows)

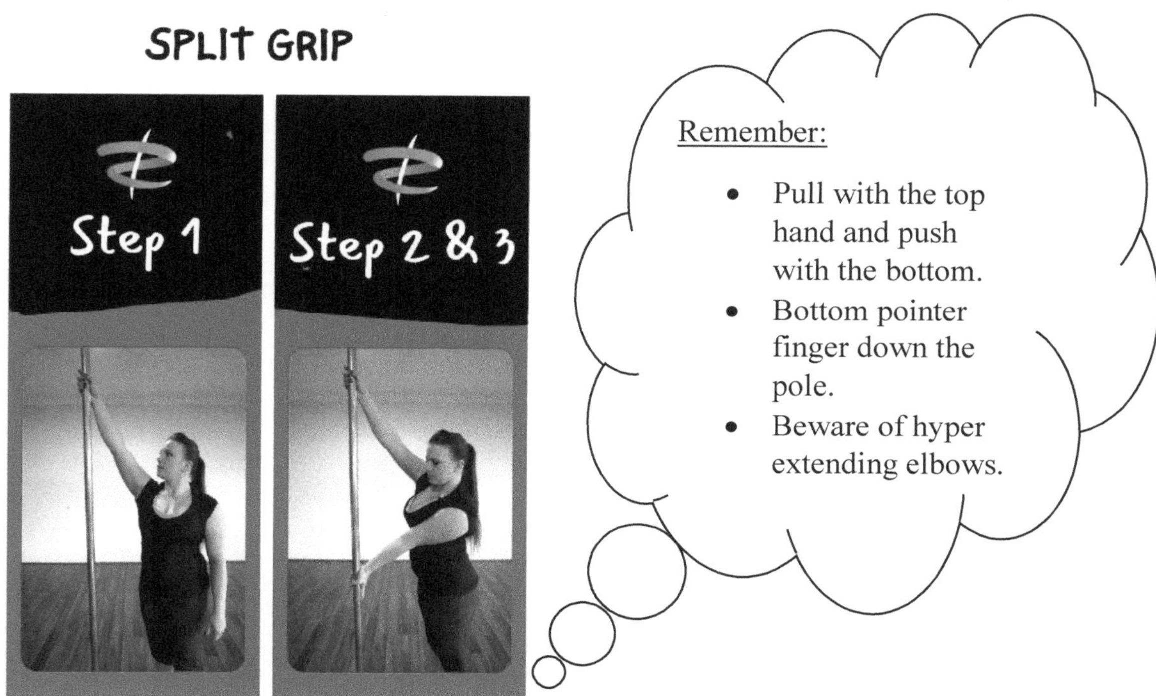

Split grip is generally used for leg-off-the-pole moves. **Basic spin grip** is great for natural flow in and out of moves with your legs on the pole, letting you glide around the pole. **Basic spin grip** also has other moves that progress from it easier – climbs, one-handed spins, and so on.

Due to the potential for elbow strain and forearm pain, I highly recommend training this grip with an instructor who can help you with technique. It's also recommended to do this grip on a spinning or unlocked pole. If you're having a fatigued or slippery day, swap back to a **forearm grip**. That way, you can still train the moves you like but with less risk to your wrists and elbows.

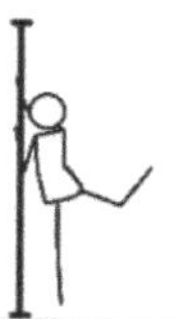

Now it's time to focus on your legs as you push and pull with your arms. Breaking it down like this gives you time to ensure that your arms are straight, your elbow is aligned, and your finger is down before spinning. It also allows you to smoothly walk into the grip and subsequent spins without feeling like there's a blockade in front of you.

When coming out of split grip, be wary not to just drop down out of it. Many people tend to release their pull from the top hand, this overloads the bottom arm and can produce forearm pain. Release your grip evenly, by placing your legs down first.

The Split Grip Fireman Spin

The first spin you're going to do in **split grip** is your **fireman**, as it gives you time to focus on your arms while your legs already know what they're doing. You also have your inside-foot behind the pole which initially puts less pressure on the grip whilst you get used to it. It doesn't shift your centre of gravity at all, giving you time to focus on this new element. One adjustment you do need to make is to hook your ankles more than your calf. Otherwise, you'll have a squashed bottom hand between your knees. By hooking your ankles, you can bring your knees out and make this spin look more pixie-like. This is the first stage of removing the reliance on your legs and transferring it to your arms and shoulders. If you point your toes, you'll notice an almost pole-sized hook behind your heel. This helps in this spin.

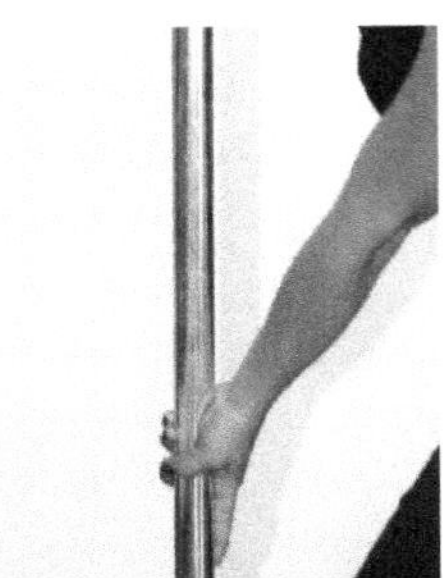

Let's have a look.

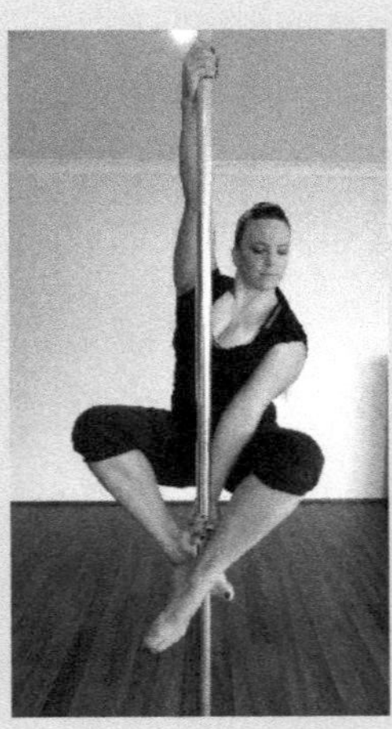

Step 1: Roll your shoulder back. Place your inside hand up, palm facing the direction you're going.

Step 2: Step on your inside leg. Pivot to face the pole.

Step 3: Place your outside hand on the pole with your finger pointing down.

Step 4: Bring your outside leg around in front of the pole, tapping your ankle onto the pole. Pull with your top arm; push with your bottom arm.

Step 5: Tap your other leg to the back of the pole. Spin!

Don't forget to practise both sides, and don't rush it. Take one step at a time. Solidify the grip, then the legs.

You now know the basics with this move, but **split grip** is such an important grip to get right, so I think it's worth a QR code, don't you? Getting a solid and safe foundation here will save a lot of stress and pain later, so watch the video!

Muscles/Areas to Strengthen for the Split Grip Fireman

- Hip flexors
- Shoulder girdle and scapular stabilisers (trapezius, serratus anterior)
- Rotator cuff (teres minor, infraspinatus)
- Abdominals (and the rest of your core, including pelvic floor)
- Forearm flexors
- Elbow stability muscles (if hyper-extensive in the elbows)

Muscles to Stretch for the Split Grip Fireman:

- Glutes
- Adductors
- Hip flexors

VISUALISATION: SPLIT GRIP FIREMAN

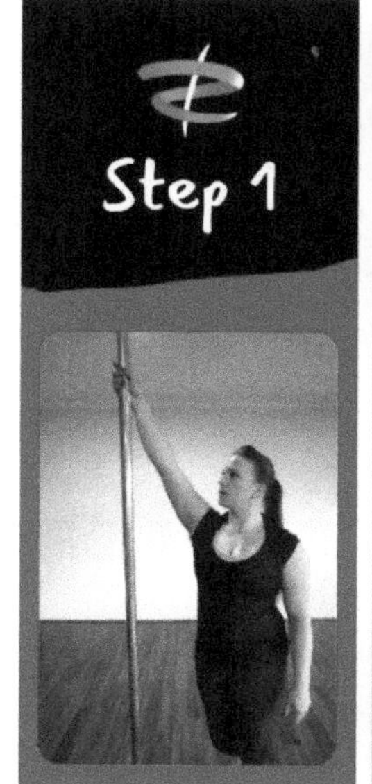

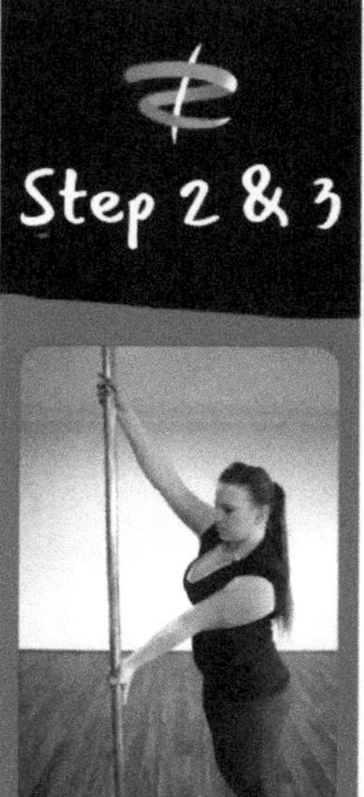

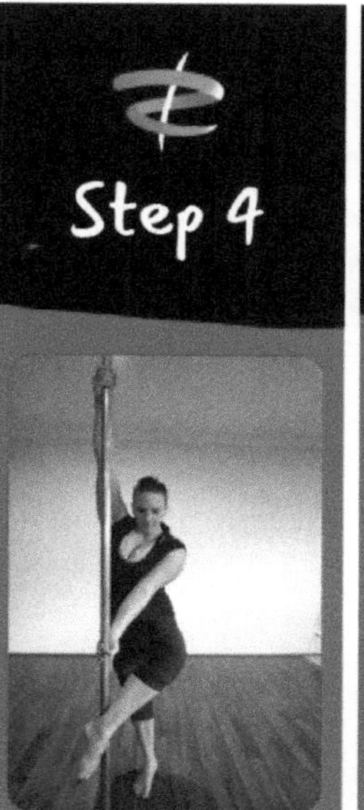

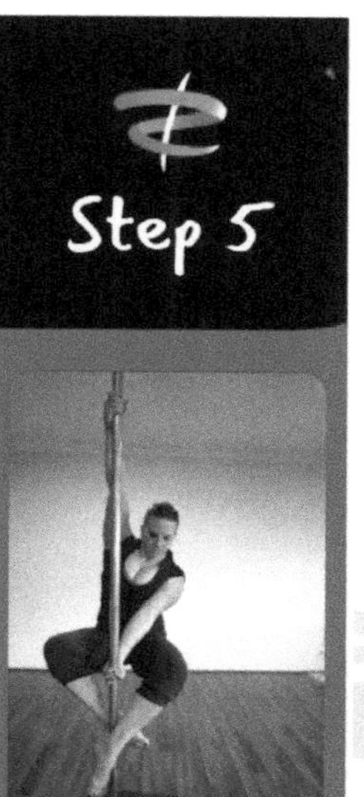

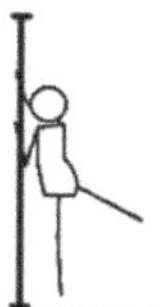

The Martini Spin

While you're focused on this grip, let's try it again, this time changing up the legs. You're going to try the **martini spin**. I find this is a favourite of many, probably because of its name. It keeps the same body alignment you've done so far, but it removes the reliance on the legs.

With the **martini spin**, you have 2 leg options. You can either slide your leg down the side of the pole or tuck that foot under your bottom. If it's floating somewhere in between, it looks like you're doing it wrong and takes away from the lines of the move.

The leg height of this one doesn't come automatically, so first, you need to focus on getting your legs into position, ensuring your knees end up next to each other, not staggered. If this is at a downwards angle to begin with, that's fine. Once the legs know what they're doing, you can start activating your abs and quads to lift your legs up in line with your hips.

Set this move just like your **fireman**: outside leg first. But this one, stays straight. Your inside leg should tap next to the pole or under your bottom. Flexing your foot around the pole is natural when you get started; the foot seeks the extra grip and safety net. Once you've gotten used to the leg placement, unhook your foot, pointing it down the pole. Flexing is a bad habit to get into and looks messy!

Take it step by step.

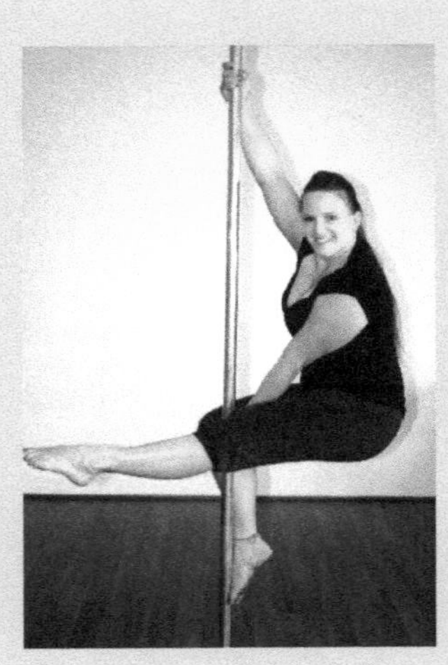

Step 1: Roll your shoulders back. Place your inside hand up, palm facing the direction you're going.

Step 2: Step on your inside leg. Pivot to face the pole.

Step 3: Place your outside hand on the pole with your finger pointing down the pole.

Step 4: Bring your outside leg around in front of the pole, keeping your leg straight. Pull with your top arm; push with your bottom arm.

Step 5: Rest your other leg next to the pole on the other side, or tuck your toes under your bottom.

Don't forget to practise both sides. Solidify your grip, then place your legs. Remember, as you're trying to start relying more on your arms, you'll need to activate your abdominals, hip flexors, and quadriceps to keep your legs up. Your legs will be lower when you first start. Don't stress about their height. Get the correct placement, practise, and then start working on the lift of your legs.

Muscles/Areas to Strengthen for the Martini Spin

- Hip flexors
- Shoulder girdle and scapular stabilisers (trapezius, serratus anterior)
- Rotator cuff (teres minor, infraspinatus)
- Adductors
- Forearm flexors
- Elbow stability muscles (if hyper-extensive in the elbows)
- Core (abs, back, and pelvic floor)

Muscles to Stretch for the Martini Spin

- Glutes
- Hamstrings

VISUALISATION: MARTINI SPIN

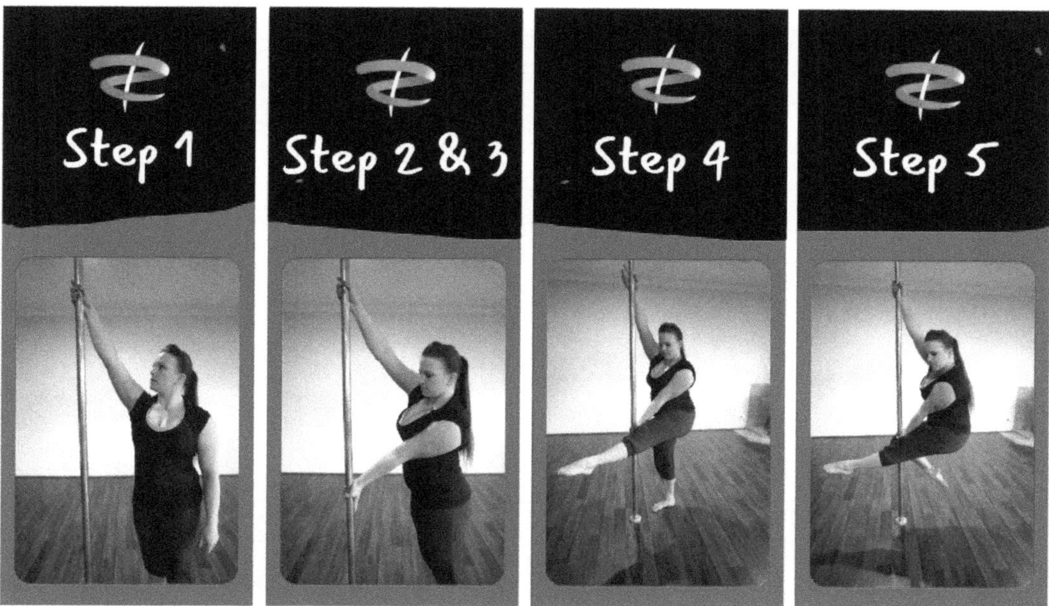

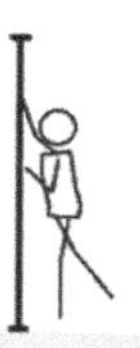

Windmill- Floor Work

There's one more pole move I suggest looking at for now. It's a **windmill**! It looks really specky and is a lot more manageable than you might think. With this one, however, you're going to train your muscle memory on the floor first. You're going to teach your legs what they're doing and warm up your joints before moving up the pole.

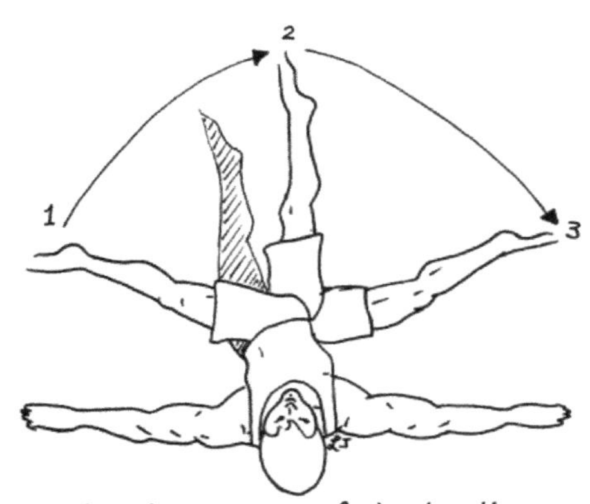

The three steps of the leading leg in the Windmill (fan kick)

Starting on your back on the floor, lift one leg up and bring it straight across your body. Then move it up so that your toes point to the roof. Next, open the leg out to the side. You should have drawn a semicircle across your body with your foot. And again. Across your body, to the sky, and out to the side.

Next, get the other leg to join in. Kick your first leg across your body, then to the sky, and while that leg is up, bring your other leg out sideways to where the first leg started. Use it to follow the first leg.

As you move your leading leg from the sky out to the side, your second (following) leg should point to the sky, then to the side, across your body, like it's following/completing the rainbow your first leg has made. You may feel like you're in a really awkward knot. Roll onto your stomach. Finish the move, and it will click.

Are you ready?

Step 1: Kick across your body.

Step 2: Circle your leg to the roof as you bring your other leg out to the side.

Step 3: Bring your first leg out to the side as the other follows to the roof, then to the side.

Step 4: Follow the momentum, and roll onto your belly.

When I roll, I tend to bend a knee. Aesthetically, it looks nicer, and it provides an easy lever to work with.

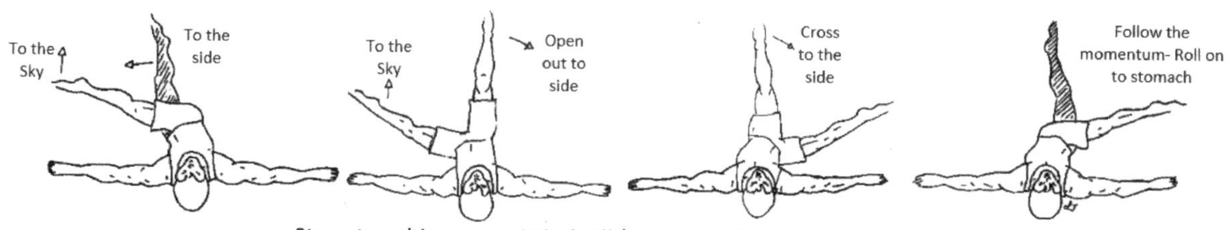

Steps to achieve your Windmill (or Fan Kick) on the floor.

This is your **windmill** on the floor. You can do it on your back or resting on your elbows. It's an awesome move. If you get stuck with the pole between your legs, you can **windmill** out. You can do it in floor routines to give your muscles a break. Adding floorwork combined with on-the-pole work creates a more dynamic, engaging routine, as not everything is at the same level.

Now that you have the flow of this, your legs know what they're doing. One is naturally following the other. It's time to move it up the pole. Holy crumble berries! I know, right? But it isn't as bad as it sounds.

Basic Invert Grip

First, you need to learn a new grip: your **basic invert grip**. No, you're not going upside down; don't stress!

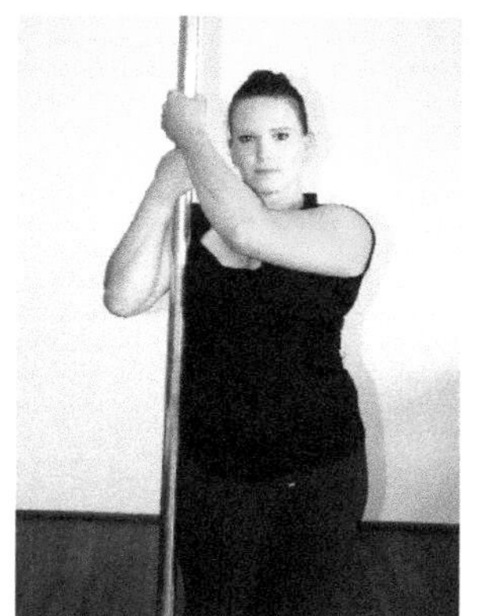

For your **basic invert grip**, stand right next to the pole, up close, with your inside arm wrapped around the pole, holding on at chin height, and your elbow pointing down. Place your outside hand just above, also at face height. You may notice from here that you can squeeze down with your inside arm and have extra grip along your bicep.

If your hands are up higher, it requires more muscle and more lift to bring your torso into the move. That isn't what you want to achieve for this move. The idea here is that you're stabilising your torso, not lifting it. Keeping your hands at head height saves all that lift and strain!

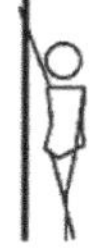

Step 1: Wrap your inside arm around the pole, holding on at face height, and keep your elbow down.

Step 2: Place your outside hand also at face height.

Step 3: Squeeze your inside arm onto the pole.

This grip can be a little uncomfortable for larger-chested people. In this situation, you may raise your outside hand higher on the pole to give your chest some space. If you do this, it's important to keep your shoulders down. Thinking of rolling them back and down helps. As long as you are within your limits and abilities, with your shoulders are engaged, they are protecting your body to keep you safe.

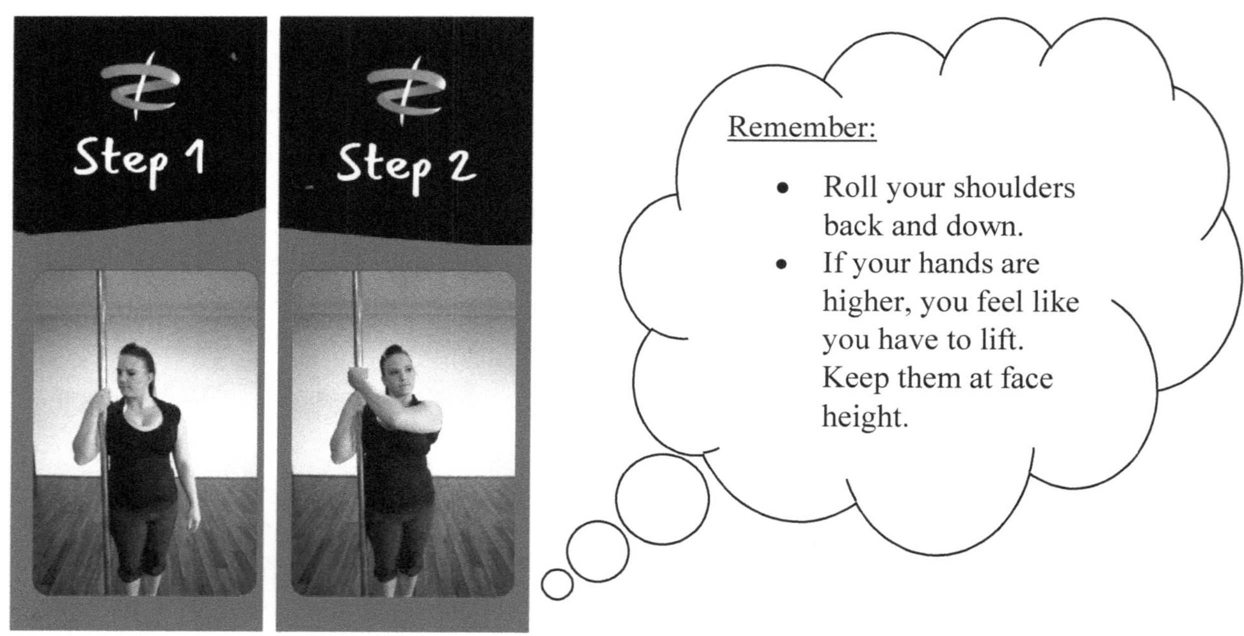

Muscles/Areas to Strengthen for the Basic Invert Grip

- Scapular stabilisers (trapezius, serratus anterior)
- Latissimus dorsi

Let's practise this grip a little. Place your hands in your **basic invert grip**, and bring your hips in front of the pole. You'll find that there is a soft, squishy spot between the rib cage and the hip bone, which is generally where the pole ends up resting.

Squeeze your bottom arm onto the pole, gripping with your top arm. Bring one knee up off the ground. Can you now swap them, bringing the other knee up as you place the first back down? And swap back again? If this is easy, can you do a swap in the air without touching the ground in between? Or bring both knees to your belly in a tuck? These are all great prep exercises to train every session!

Now, as long as you weren't dropping down into your arms during the above exercises, you're ready to try the **windmill (also known as fan kick) on the pole.**

Windmill (or Fan Kick) on the pole

You've set your hands in your **basic invert grip**. Remember, the idea is to stabilise your body while your head and shoulders stay still (you aren't lifting yourself up!). Let's look at the rest of your body.

Kick your inside leg out, away from the pole, at a 45-degree angle. This brings your hips in front of the pole. Trust me: you don't want to slam your hip bone into a pole! Now circle your inside leg around in front of the pole to land on the other side. Your second leg will follow. That's why you always practise on the ground first, not only to warm up the joints but also to show your second leg what to do.

Once you've circled one leg, then the other leg, you'll land twisted. This is where the roll from the floor comes in handy. However, you're now standing. Pivot on the ball of your foot to face the pole. This finishes the move and makes you feel like you've done it. Without the twist, you won't feel like you're achieving; it's all in the pivot! Sometimes initially it feels like a "step..step.. pivot" – it will get there with practice!

Don't worry about the height of your legs. Start off low, and get used to the motion. As you practise, you'll notice that your legs will come up higher. Once you're comfortable in the grip, you can activate your abs and quads more to create a lift. You can also tilt slightly back in the torso when you have more grip control. This gives the illusion of height when flexibility isn't what it appears.

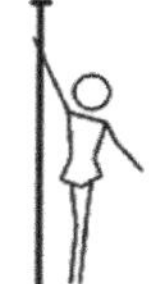

Let's break it down

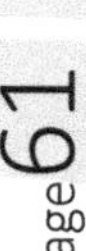

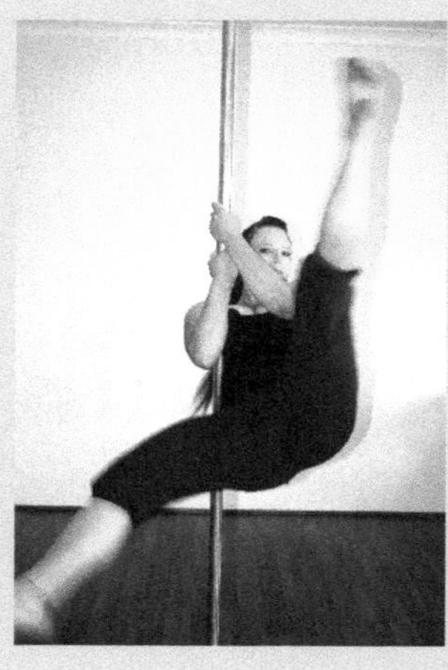

Step 1: Wrap your inside arm around the pole, holding on at face height, with your elbow down.

Step 2: Place your outside hand at face height.

Step 3: Squeeze your inside arm onto the pole.

Step 4: Take a small step with your outside leg so that you can kick your inside leg away from the pole to bring the hip in front.

Step 5: Circle your inside leg around towards the pole and down the other side. The other leg should follow.

Step 6: Pivot to face the pole.

You can do this with a little pivot and go the other way, or you can do it again and again, constantly around the pole. Don't forget to train both sides.

At this point, I suggest also practising getting into the spins you have learnt so far. Can you get into them from a walk? How can you swoop your legs out and around to create momentum? Play with your style until you're able to pole walk into the moves you've done so far. Put on some music, and have some fun with it!

This one is a lot of fun, but it's also a whole new way of moving. A QR code may help you out. Let the video guide you and help with your flow.

Muscles/Areas to Strengthen for the Windmill

- Scapular stabilisers (trapezius, serratus anterior)
- Latissimus dorsi
- Abdominals (and the rest of your core too!)
- Hip flexors

Muscles to Stretch for the Windmill

- Glutes
- Hamstrings

VISUALISATION: WINDMILL

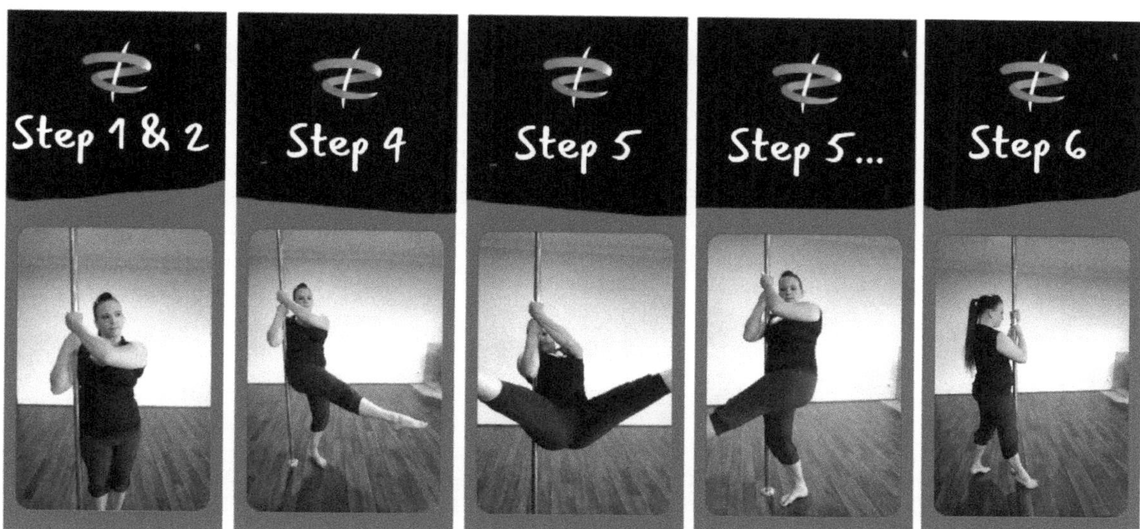

Please be aware of your resting training habits, things like sticking your tongue out when you concentrate or biting your lip are not recommended. If you do these, I highly suggest making a conscious effort to stop before you accidentally cause an injury. Remember to always breathe through your exercises.

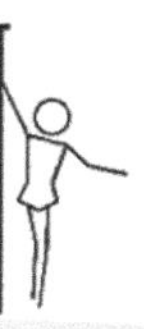

Putting Moves Together

By now, you have enough moves to play with to create small routines. There are lots of transitions, fake spins, step-arounds, dip spins, twirls, and pirouettes, even classic hip circles, chest circles, and body rolls. That's without delving into the world of walks and floor moves.

I'm not here to put my style onto you. Don't feel restricted by how you 'should' move. Make it your own. Choose your own music and your own style of movement... I'm just here to help you learn technical pole spins and get them done safely. In saying that, learning a few combinations is helpful on your journey, so let's have a look.

Pole Pirouette

Try the **back-to-pole pirouette** to change directions. If you don't want to change directions, once your back is to the pole, add in a cheeky kick and slide down to the floor. Just make sure that your grounded foot is far enough forward that your knee never goes over your toes as you descend!

The pirouette motion is great to get used to, as it will help a lot of other moves, pirouettes, and transitions make more sense.

You can step your back straight to the pole, or you can spin under your arm to get there. This move allows you to go up, down, left, or right. You can even add a pose or dance break! I set my feet at the end (step 5 below), as it helps you to ground and regain balance, especially if you are wearing shoes. Also, having a slight bend in your knees helps you feel stable at the end and helps with the dizzies.

Step 1: Hold on to the pole with your inside hand up high and your shoulders rolled back.

Step 2: Step on your outside leg towards the front of the pole.

Step 3: Pivot on the ball of your outside foot to face the pole, going under your top arm.

Step 4: Keep pivoting until you can rest your back on the pole.

Step 5: Put your inside foot down, pointing your outside foot (step, point).

If you're in heels and that little roll at the toe is throwing you off balance slightly, try using your hands to stabilise.

Step 1: Hold on to the pole with your inside hand up high and your shoulders rolled back.

Step 2: Step in front of the pole on your outside leg. Bring your outside hand to the pole on the same side as your body. Push the pole gently away with your little finger to assist the turn.

Step 3: Pivot to face the pole, going under your top arm. As you turn, roll your hand so your thumb faces down. This way, you can grab the pole.

Step 4: Keep going until you can rest your back on the pole.

Step 5: Put your inside foot down, pointing your outside foot.

Following these steps, you'll have finished with one hand up on the pole and one down behind your back, almost forming an S shape. It looks nice and creates a balanced shape, which helps you balance too.

Fireman-to-backward spin

Now for the **fireman-to-backward spin**! The hardest thing about this one is overthinking because you're suddenly going backward without changing direction. Let's have a look.

Here goes the **fireman**.

Step 1: Place your inside hand up, palm facing the direction you're going. Roll your shoulders back.

Step 2: Place your outside hand across your body, holding on at chest height.

Step 3: Step onto your inside leg to bring your outside leg in front of the pole (knee on one side, ankle on the other).

Step 4: Tap your other leg to the back of the pole (knee on one side, ankle on the other so that one knee is on each side of the pole).

Step 5: Pop your toes on the ground, following the direction of the momentum of the spin. Pivot on the ball of your foot under your top arm.

Step 6: Pick up your now outside leg, and draw it out in a wide circle. Now you're starting your **backward-knees position**! If you need to raise onto your tippy-toes, allow your hands to slide higher up the pole before spinning, or you may end up too close to the ground.

Step 7: Draw a circle going behind you with your outside leg.

Step 8: As your calf touches the pole, bend your knees.

Step 9: Spin, gravity helping you down to the ground!

Sound a little confusing? Now that you've heard the long-winded version, a quick recap should make sense.

Land on your tippy-toes, and push up to restraighten your body. Keep momentum going in the same direction. Pivot under your top arm (don't move your hands). Now pick up your outside leg, and draw your circle to spin into your **backward-knees position**.

Front-knee-hook to back-knee-hook

This move is commonly known as **forward knees to backward knees**. This one is fab because your body does all the work naturally, though it may stop halfway if the momentum isn't there. This move is so much fun! Again, it's just allowing the flow. All you need to think about is unhooking your inside leg. The body naturally unwinds to face the other way, and then there is the panic to hook the leg on the pole. If you don't have enough momentum, your body will unwind to face the pole. Try with a bit more oomph in the spin and see the difference!

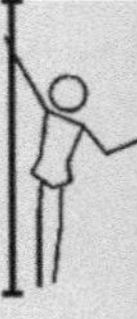

Step 1: Place your inside hand up, palm facing the direction you're going. Roll your shoulders back.

Step 2: Place your outside hand across your body, holding on at chest height.

Step 3: Bend your inside leg onto the pole.

Step 4: Raise up on the ball of your outside foot.

Step 5: Lean forward through your hips, bending the other leg when you need to. Let gravity do the work!

Step 6: Once you've made it halfway around the pole, unhook your leg and re-hook the leg that's now closest to the pole. The body naturally pivots in the middle. Just keep your bent knee position in the air, and let it flow.

Step 7: Spin down to the ground.

Just remember: unhook, re-hook. You've got this!

While we are looking at going backwards; try pivoting under the arm to a **back-knee hook** (backward knees). You don't always have to do an obvious turn to get into a backward spin. Making it flow can gain extra momentum for you and be a lot of fun. Going backward from a walk sounds tricky, but the pivots are fab!

Step 1: Go for your walk with your shoulders rolled back. Place your inside hand up, palm facing the direction you're going.

Step 2: Step onto your outside leg. Pivot under your arm towards the pole. You'll notice that this arm has become your outside arm and is in the **reverse spin grip** position.

Step 3: Wrap your inside hand around the pole at shoulder height.

Step 4: Draw a circle going behind you with your outside leg. It will be a bit bigger and feel faster this time.

Step 5: As your calf touches the pole, bend your knees and spin.

With some spins, it can seem trickier to create flow, as you start in a static position. The knee-hook spins (forward and backward) are definitely some of these. But it is possible to step in and out of them to create flow, not always heading to the ground. Let's learn to step in and out of the **front-knee hook** (forward knees).

The trick to stepping out of all spins is to allow your body to follow the flow of the momentum. With **forward and backward knees**, your body is quite close to the pole, so this is easier, but with other spins, you may need to lean your hips out to allow the momentum to flow while keeping the alignment of your body. Otherwise, you may be tempted to pull yourself upright with your arm, and this will stop the flow of momentum, as it will change the direction of your pull on the pole. Technical stuff, but when you work it out, things feel so much smoother!

If you go for a walk around the pole, ensuring your shoulders are set and rolled back, you can do a big flair with your inside leg. By flair, I mean kicking in forward and bringing your outside leg around, letting some of your body weight travel with it as you go onto the ball of your foot. Bend your inside leg at the usual spot around the pole as you grab on with your outside hand and use that momentum to spin.

To come out of this spin without going to the ground, place the ball of your inside foot on the floor. Then bring your outside leg around to join it. This flair around the outside leg looks very pretty if you can straighten it as it comes around. You'll almost finish like you're sitting in a pretend chair. You can body roll out of this and continue or, eventually, walk straight out of the move.

Again?

Step 1: Walk with your shoulders rolled back and your inside hand up high.

Step 2: Bring your inside leg forward and around.

Step 3: Bend your inside leg onto the pole as you grab on with your outside hand.

Step 4: Pick up your other foot to spin.

Step 5: Place your inside toes down on the ground.

Step 6: Bring your outside leg around, pivoting to end with feet together.

(false) Step-around Spin

False step-arounds are a fun way of gaining momentum, allowing for all sorts of smooth grip changes. **False step-arounds** look like a spin, though they are not. They give the illusion of more effort being put in. Really, your arms just need those few seconds of rest! The theory behind the **false step-around** is that with your hand up high, you take a step with your outside foot and let your grip and body move around the pole so that your step lands right next to the other foot. It's like taking an almost 360-degree step. Try the **false step-around** to **back-knee hook**.

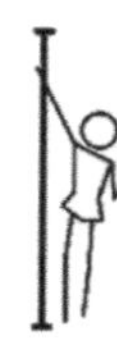

Step 1: Go for your walk with your shoulders rolled back and your inside hand up, palm facing the direction you're going.

Step 2: Step on your inside leg.

Step 3: Bring your outside leg in a big step around the pole, placing it back next to your inside leg. Stay on the ball of your foot.

Step 4: Pivot under your arm towards the pole. You'll notice that this arm has become your outside arm and is in the **reverse spin grip** position.

Step 5: Wrap your inside hand around the pole at shoulder height.

Step 6: Draw a circle going behind you with your outside leg. It will be a bit bigger and feel faster this time.

Step 7: As your calf touches the pole, bend your knees and spin.

This is very similar to the **dip-spin**, where you bend your knees, bringing your bottom back as you step around. However, with the dip-spin you lose the momentum and the ability to flow as easily into other moves. In saying that, the dip-spin is a nice move and really plays with bodies curves.

Pivot Turns

Now for **body roll pivot turns**! Your body roll can feel totally disjointed. Think of it like you're a giant tongue licking a pole. First, your nose goes to the pole, then your chest, then your belly button. Then you sink back into your hips. If your knees are slightly bent and your feet staggered, you'll find that fluidity comes a lot easier. Now you can use this move to change directions. If you face the side of the pole, feet staggered with one in front, one behind, and knees soft, pretend you're a tongue going in to lick the side of the pole (use your inside hand to hold the pole for stability). Your nose, chest, and belly will sink deeper back into your hips.

Now draw a semicircle with your hips while all your weight is back there. Pivot on the ball of your foot, and turn to face the other way. Swap hands, and do it again. Nose, chest, belly button, sink into your hips, pivot as you drag your bottom back and around in a C shape, and you're back. Swap hands.

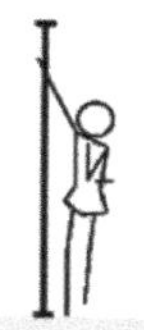

This way, you can change direction so that your other hand is on top without anyone knowing that was what you were doing. It smooths that moment of 'I want to do this spin, but I can only do it on the dodgy side'. It allows you to incorporate the move into routines. It also gives your arms a break from holding up your body weight!

Step 1: Place your nose forward (side on to the pole).
Step 2: Use your chest to follow.
Step 3: Follow with your belly button.
Step 4: Sink back into your hips.
Step 5: Pivot to the other side, and swap hands.
Step 6: Repeat.

Star (Jazzy) Side Steps

Not feeling body rolls to change directions? They aren't your only option. **Star sidesteps** can be really jazzy. Stand side on to the pole, arms and legs out like a star, holding on to the pole with your inside hand. Step towards the pole with your outside leg, and bring your outside hand to the pole, almost like you're going to hug the pole. Open up as a star on the other side, letting go of the first hand and stepping out. Suddenly, you're on the other side of the pole with the other hand on the pole. Just like turning the page of a book; open, close, and open on the other side.

This can be awkward, so what I do is plant my outside leg on the floor. I put all my weight on this outside leg and point the toe of the inside leg, bringing my arm up on a diagonal. This gives pretty lines and makes the move look a lot more dramatic. By having your weight on the outside leg, you'll have set yourself up for your next move. You can take a step on your inside leg without having to play around with transferring your weight. Once you get the flow of it, it's a lot of fun.

Step 1: Hold on with your inside hand, body out like a star.
Step 2: Step to the pole with your outside leg.
Step 3: Swap hands to hold on with the other hand.
Step 4: Open out again on the other side of the pole, transferring weight and pointing the inside toe (step, point).
Step 5: Now add your spin of choice on the other side!

Have a play. Try putting the moves you've learnt into different combinations. Getting fluidity in the moves you know helps to get your body used to them dynamically. You can do an awesome cardio routine and really get to know how you move with and around the pole. Everything makes more sense if you know how the moves work and flow. Have some fun! Put your favourite music on, and play.

The kick and slide can be a fun transitional move to get you from standing to down the pole. With your back to the pole, you can do all sorts of hair flicks, chest bumps, hip figure eights, and other dance-like moves while giving your arms a rest.

Still not up to more spins? Head to the ground! Stagger your feet in front of you so that when you squat down, your knees don't go over your toes. Find a comfy spot on your back to press back into the pole (still rather central but off to one side). If you go on the soft/squishy bit of your shoulder, you can play with different head positionings more easily. Push back onto the pole as you slide to squat down. This way, you don't have to hold on, and you still have support. Alternatively, hold above your head for dramatic pose purposes (and support).

You can squat down from here into a position to do little **bunny squats** (bounces) or **peek-a-boos** (spreading knees apart and together). Alternatively, you can kick one leg before you squat and slide down. You'll end up on your bottom in a posed sit. This is an easier doorway to floor moves.

This is also a good conditioning move. If you put your foot back on the floor before you go lower than 90 degrees with your thighs, push against the pole with your back, and slide back up. Kick the other leg, slide to 90 degrees, place your foot down, and push to slide back up.

Placing your feet down, and the way you do it can really assist your flow. Having one foot pointed, with the weight on the other foot allows for the pointed foot to be the next step. Maintaining the transitional movements on the balls of your feet allows you to pivot and create flow easier, than if you were flat footed.

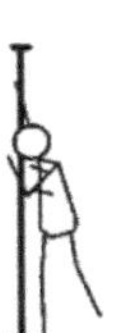

One big thing is to feel the flow of the momentum, the big round swoops of your leg, as you create a straight line from your top hand all the way down to the toes, it helps you feel more locked in and secure in your movement; in saying that you need to know where you are going to place your limbs next. You can listen to the beats of your favourite music, and just move to the music without overthinking it. Slow moves down, don't rush them, a good tip is to hold each move (especially on spin pole) for a count of 3 before looking at transitioning to the next move. I personally like to pick my favourite three moves and work out different ways of putting them together. Then once three becomes easy, I pick five moves, and practice different transitions in and out, even mixing up the order of the moves. If you are on the floor, you can pick a letter, find different ways to trace that letter on the floor with your body.

Focusing on how different musical tracks make you feel and moving in those emotions is a great start finding your flow, find a song that makes you happy, sad, angry, sexy, and flow with it. Move with the song, and your body, not your head, don't get lost in thoughts (unless it is of safety). You can even focus on dynamic levels, have and up movement, followed by a down movement, then back up again, even if that is just a hand or a leg creating the up/down movement. We fly on pole, so we want to create that link between the sky and the earth. Create a relationship with your pole- why is it there, what is its purpose, bring that emotion and feeling, that relationship into your routine. It isn't there for you to just spin on… what is its reason for existing in that space? What link do you have to the pole, explore that link. It doesn't have to be about tricks, they come with time and practice, your flow and ability to create your own style of movement comes from within.

There can be so much emotion in putting together a routine, but there is also a lot of technicalities about how to link moves, and create that flow, more so once the moves get more advanced. The *"Personal Pole and Aerial Record,"*[23] as much as it is a planner more than anything, has a small section on transitions and looking at where your contact points are to help you work out where your next move can flow from. It talks about linking moves with the same contact points; between your body and the pole, understanding this really helps create flow and allows you to really understand the movements and transitions. Which, in turn, makes it easier to choreograph and plan a routine.

Getting Up Off the Floor

You've gotten down to the ground a few times now, clambering your way back up. Now it's time to practise and get in the habit of getting up nicely every time! It is such a good and important habit to get into. Getting up smoothly, nicely, is not only good practice for technique and control, but totally empowering too. Feeling graceful, sometimes even sensual, about the way that you get up and move. It really helps to finish things off and make you feel the flow.

Peek-a-boo

One option is to **peek-a-boo** to standing. This gives you the option to push yourself up to standing without it looking like you're struggling to get up. This, however, doesn't work if your legs are wrapped around the pole, so you may have to crawl away to do this one. Let's have a look at how it works.

Starting on your knees, transfer your body weight forward onto them so that you can tuck your toes under your bottom. Now transfer your weight back onto the balls of your feet and balance. You're now in a squat position.

Pop your hands on your thighs, just above your knees, as if you were going to press down to stand up. But that's not very elegant. Instead, be cheeky. Push your knees open and out to the side, then close them again. Now push on your thighs as you roll up, head first, and slide your hands up your legs as you go. You're now using your body to help with momentum as you rise up.

Step 1: Kneel down.
Step 2: Transfer your weight onto your knees.
Step 3: Tuck your toes under your bottom.
Step 4: Rock back to a squat.
Step 5: Place your hands just above your knees.
Step 6: Open and close your legs.
Step 7: Roll up, pressing on your legs for initial leverage.

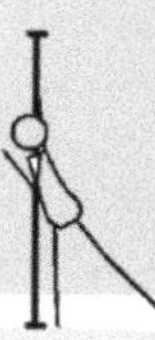

This is a great move to help you start to get up. But if you're wrapped around the pole, it's a tad tricky. In that case, I would think of creating **tripods** to help stand. This can be as dramatic as you choose to make it.

Tripod to stand

Start on your knees with the pole between your legs as if you have just done a **knee-hook spin**. Place your hands on the floor in front of you at around shoulder height. Jump your legs forward in front of the pole. With your legs straight and your hands on the floor, you have created your first **tripod**. You'll notice that there is such a thing as too big or too small of a jump. This comes down to your personal balance point, which you'll need to find. You want to be able to lean back and rest your bottom on the pole comfortably.

With your bottom on the pole, you can remove your hands from the floor. You've created your second **tripod**! Now roll up, face first, like a dramatic body roll. I like to drag my hands up my legs slowly as I roll up too.

Let's break it down.

Step 1: Kneel down with the pole between your legs.
Step 2: Place your hands on the floor at around shoulder height.
Step 3: Jump to straight legs a little bit in front of the pole (**tripod 1**).
Step 4: Lean back until your bottom touches the pole (**tripod 2**).
Step 5: Lift your head up, and roll to stand.

If you're in heels, the roll forward over the toe part of the shoe can be tricky, but with some balanced and purposeful hand placement, you can resolve this issue.

Are you ready?

Step 1: Kneel down with the pole between your legs.
Step 2: Place your hands on the floor at around shoulder height.
Step 3: Jump to straight legs in front of the pole (**tripod 1**).
Step 4: Lean back until your bottom touches the pole (**tripod 2**).
Step 5: Place one hand on the pole between your legs.
Step 6: Lift your head as you commence your roll up. Place your other hand on the pole at your lower back.
Step 7: Continue your roll up, placing the hand that was between your legs over your head. And pose!

The great thing about doing it like this is that the 3 steps create a good flow balance, using purposeful movements that provide drama and stability. It's like a 1, 2, 3. BAM! You land posed, left and right balanced, with both arms on the pole almost in an S shape.

Side Body Rolls

Side body rolls are also fun if you're close to the pole without your legs hooked. They're smooth and dancey, just rolling! **Side body rolls** flow best from a squat. I've included the steps to get into a squat, but if you're already there, don't change anything!

Step 1: Kneel down.
Step 2: Transfer your weight to your knees.
Step 3: Tuck your toes under your bottom.
Step 4: Rock back to a squat.
Step 5: Pivot to side on, and bring your inside hand to the pole, placing your outside hand on your leg, just above your knee.
Step 6: Body roll up, bottom up and roll. Pull on the pole and press on your legs for initial leverage.

Triangle Slides

Triangle slides are another good option to stand. You can slow down to allow for extra dramatics and stabilisation.

Step 1: Start in a squat.
Step 2: Jump/slide one leg out straight to the side.
Step 3: Look up, hands on your thighs.
Step 4: Push down on your bent leg to ground yourself as you slide to stand (pull with your adductors).
Step 5: Slide your outer leg in to bring your legs together.

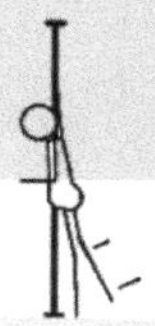

Dramatic moves. Eat your heart out! And strut!

There are many more ways to get up off the floor. These are my go-to moves! Feel free to play and find your own. Use purposeful, balanced movements with specific hand positions so that you don't look like you're flailing, and make it your own!

Low-Lift Step Around

The **low-lift fireman prep/step-around** is also a fun move to play with, especially with a shorter pole. Let's start nice and low, squatting on the floor. Hold on to the pole in your **basic spin grip**, and step to the other side of the pole. Rock from one side to the other, getting used to the motion.

Now try again. Step to the other side, rock, and use that momentum to stand up. Pretty simple, right? Simple but messy! Let's pretty up your legs!

Squat down again, and bring your outside leg out to your side, posed and straight. Now drag that leg out in a circle to the other side of the pole. Here goes the momentum rock and stand! Drag your inside leg in as you stand up. Have a few goes at this to get the motion on both sides. Later, you can use this motion and turn it into a spin.

When I spin, I prefer **split grip** so that I have space to see where I can place my legs. Otherwise, I feel a bit crowded.

Let's take a look.

Step 1: Squat down, facing the pole.

Step 2: Place your outside leg out to your side.

Step 3: Place your inside hand up, palm facing the direction you're going. Roll your shoulder back.

Step 4: Stretch your outside hand across your body, holding on to the pole at chest height as you slide your outside leg in a circle to the other side of the pole.

Step 5: Follow the momentum to stand on the other leg, dragging your feet in.

VISUALISATION: LOW-LIFT FIREMAN PREP

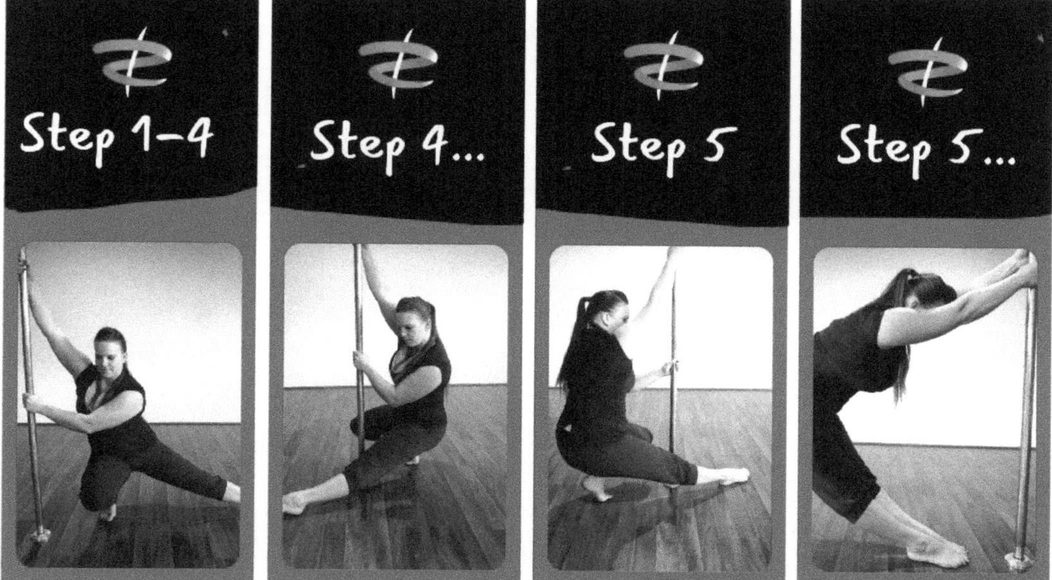

Getting Dizzy

As we've already covered, spinning poles allow for more mistakes. Your alignment can be out, and you will still spin, so it's important to be precise with your movements. In the end, it requires more muscle and control to be balanced and achieve safely. Go static first with all new moves. This makes sure that you have the mechanics of the move right. If you're not aligned and activating the right muscles, the move won't work. Once you know you're strong, safe, and balanced, move to spin, and practise different speeds and modifications.

What if you're on a static pole but STILL get dizzy? We've all seen the dodgy old-school dinosaur movies, yeah? A T-rex is coming. There's a puddle of water. Each step the T-rex takes: BOOM! The puddle ripples. The same thing applies here.

When you're dizzy, all the liquid in your ear is swirling around like a whirlpool. A solid 2-foot jump goes boom onto the floor like a T-rex step. That liquid stops spinning, it ripples out and settles. Dizziness, be gone! Seriously, it's amazing!

When you're ready to give a spinning pole a go, where do you start? To be honest, I rarely use my spinning pole. I've had ear issues from birth, and since giving birth, it seems that spin affects me a lot more! I remember the very first time I found a spinning pole in 2007. I had no idea it spun. I was so excited to find somewhere new with a pole that I almost ran and leapt into a spin, and I held on tight! It just kept going!

Some moves look amazing on spinning poles, so if you're keen to give one a go, here are some pointers.

Don't jump straight into spinning. Where is your natural comfort zone for static? What is second nature? Try a few basics, then work up to your second-nature moves before trying anything tricky. Get used to how the pole works and how your body works with the pole. Static poles are a battle between momentum and body weight. Now you have to add spin. Go through each move from the basics. Your muscles aren't accustomed to stabilising. It will feel completely different here!

Use both hands! It's amazing how quickly one hand, leg, or even head position can change the spin. Start all moves with both hands, even if you can do them one-handed on a static pole. Once you're confident with how you move on the spinning pole, you can start changing these positions and try one-handed, but make sure you only change one aspect at a time to allow yourself the chance to get used to it.

Use a spotter, and make sure your spotter knows what move you're going to attempt so they know how to spot and where to stand so they don't get injured. Their job is not to lift or hold you; that's your job. The spotter is there to protect your head, neck, and back in the event of an incident. If you can't hold the move, regress it, and train the regressions more until you build up your strength.

Velocity! With spinning poles, the movement comes from a completely different set of mechanics than with a static pole. You can slightly arch your back and create spin, then pull your body in or out to change speed. Stepping into moves is enough to start the spin. Then it's about holding that position, not creating momentum to spin. Step or lean into spins. Don't throw yourself in. It's physics, just like when you were a kid and someone would spin you on a swing. When you brought your legs in, you sped up, and when you stuck a limb out, you slowed down. It's all about the path of resistance. Be aware of the height of your pole. The higher it is, the more force there will be behind your spins. Every spinning pole is a little bit different. Play within your comfort zone, trying different elements with your body. Find how movements work and how you feel with each change.

It may be worth looking at your routine, what do you need to include in your warm ups, are you holding tension in your neck and shoulders? Are you stressed and distracted? Have you got a bottle of water with you? What about your eat and sleep habits? All these can affect your bodies response to exercise.

Your body gets used to spinning. It does get easier with practice. But at the same time, if you have liquid in your ear, it spins with you. You stop, and it keeps spinning.

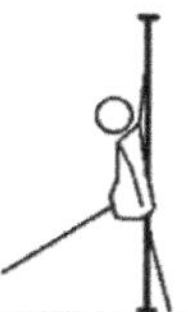

Helping Dizziness on a Spinning Pole

- Keep your head still/level. Bobbing adds to the motion. Eventually, you can play with flicks and shapes, but for now, get used to the motion. Keeping your head still also helps you maintain correct alignment.
- Look in one spot as you spin, and always go back to it. Don't watch the room swirl around you. This increases turbulence in your ear and leads to all sorts of dizziness!
- If spotting leads to a sore neck, another option is to unfocus your gaze and let your eyes flow with the motion without focusing. If you need to focus on something, focus on the pole.
- Spin in both directions, even in your routine. It's good for your muscles, and it helps to balance out your inner ear.
- Stretch your neck thoroughly (if needed) prior to a spin session. Sometimes, there's too much tension in there, and that throws you off. Please be careful with your neck. It's a fragile thing. Don't force or overdo any action (including stretching).
- Add some ginger to your drinking water. It's known to be good for nausea if this is a concern for you.

Hopefully, you'll have solved the issue. As I predominantly train on static poles, the T-rex jump is enough for me; sometimes with a few neck stretches. Everyone is different, so not all tricks to stop the "dizzies" will work for each person, it is about finding out what works for you. I bring my body out very quickly as the spinning pole spins. You can do some beautiful moves on a spinning pole, so I definitely see the appeal. Your personal preference and journey are the key. Find your own style and preferences, and be true to yourself!

Removing the Reliance on the Legs

One-Handed Fireman Spin

The **one-handed fireman** isn't as scary as it sounds! But you're going back to basics with a **basic spin grip**. Train this with your hand on the pole, slowly releasing the grip of your bottom (outside) hand, one finger at a time, until you're confident enough in your grip to release it completely.

Let's give it a go.

Step 1: Place your inside hand up the pole, palm facing the direction you're going. Roll your shoulder back to stabilise and activate the shoulder muscles.

Step 2: Stretch your outside hand across your body, holding on at chest height.

Step 3: Step on your inside leg to bring your outside leg in front of the pole (knee on one side, ankle on the other).

Step 4: Tap your other leg to the back of the pole (knee on one side, ankle on the other so that one knee is on each side of the pole).

Step 5: Spin! Test to see if you can release your fingers or even the grip of your bottom hand.

Now that you have a bit more confidence, it's actually easier with more momentum and starting with your bottom hand off. Start with it straight out to the side. Eventually, you can look at giving that hand a purpose, whether it be pointing at people, putting it on your hip, or something else. Remember, momentum is key, but please ensure that you're comfortable with your grip from the above exercise before trying this. Also keep in mind, your top hand is your "spinning hand" it is what you are rotating from- this had always stays put, do not try and remove the top hand. Ensure that you are actively pulling with the top hand, but focus on removing the bottom hand!

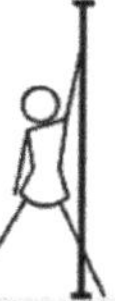

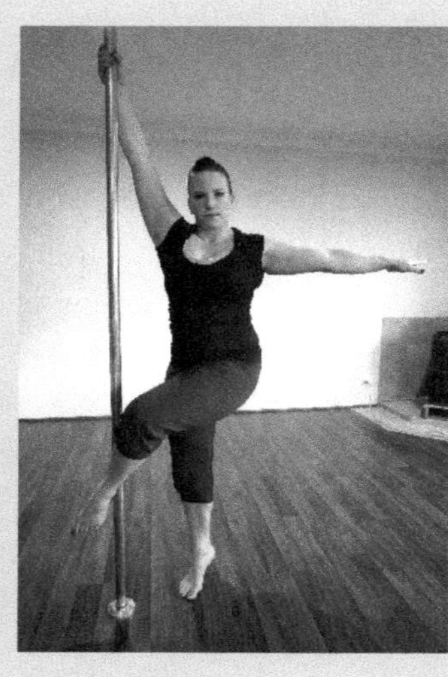

Step 1: Place your inside hand up the pole, palm facing the direction you're going. Roll your shoulder back.

Step 2: Stretch your outside hand straight out to the side in line with your shoulder.

Step 3: Step on your inside leg to bring your outside leg in front of the pole (knee on one side, ankle on the other).

Step 4: Tap your other leg to the back of the pole (knee on one side, ankle on the other so that one knee is on each side of the pole).

Step 5: Spin!

One- Handed Front-Knee Hook

The **one-handed forward knees** (aka **front-knee hook**) is a little less daunting in the way that you're using gravity, but at the same time, you can sometimes feel like you're going to faceplant if you don't line your hips up. Remember, hips first in your spin! With this one, it's easy to hang out of your shoulder, so remember to roll your shoulder back and activate it first.

Start with your outside hand off the pole this time, as bringing the hand off the pole mid-spin is going against the direction of the spin, and that throws things off. Put your hand on your hip. It can be a reminder to push through the hips first to spin.

Are you ready?

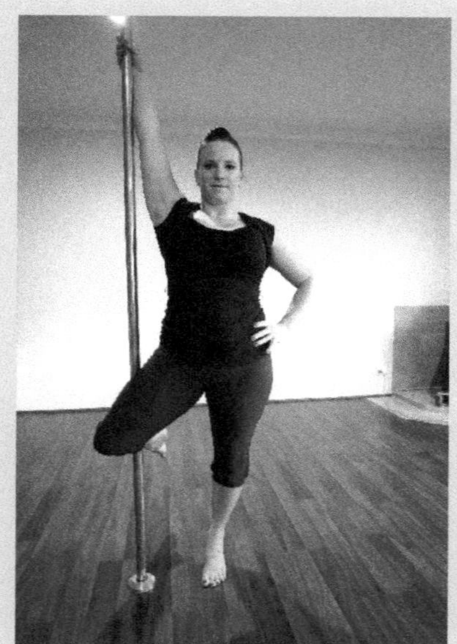

Step 1: Place your inside hand up, palm facing the direction you're going. Roll your shoulder back.

Step 2: Put your outside hand on your hip, thinking of pushing it forward.

Step 3: Bend your inside leg onto the pole.

Step 4: Stand up on the ball of your foot on your outside leg.

Step 5: Lean forward through your hips, bending your other leg when you need to. Let gravity do the work!

Step 6: Spin to the floor. Don't forget to train both sides.

Muscles/Areas to Strengthen for One-Handed Spins

These are the same as the spin themselves, but as a quick reminder, they are:

Fireman Spin:

- Hip flexors
- Shoulder girdle and scapular stabilisers (trapezius, serratus anterior)
- Rotator cuff (teres minor, infraspinatus)
- Core (abs, back, and pelvic floor)

Front Knee hook:

- Shoulder girdle and scapular stabilisers (trapezius, serratus anterior)
- Rotator cuff (teres minor, infraspinatus)
- Pectorals
- Hamstrings
- Core (including pelvic floor)

Muscles to Stretch for One-Handed Spins

- Latissimus dorsi
- Side flexors
- Pectorals

The Lift and Slide

The **pole lift and slide** isn't a move you do for the sake of moves. It's more of a move for you to do a mental check. What's your grip like? How hard is too hard or too soft to grip? This move helps you link all your little neural pathways and use that knowledge for future training. It helps you learn your comfort zones with grip and determine how much slip you can control comfortably for spins. It's also a good move to revisit on slippery days to help you work out what's a safe grip.

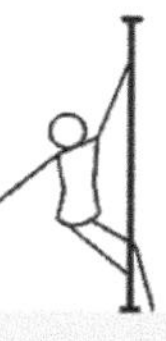

I have you landing on your knees. Unless you have knee issues, it's generally safe to land kneeling, and it makes you hold control for longer than if you released onto your feet. But if you need a mat under your knees, feel free to use one.

Basically, you're going to hold on to the pole just above face height. Lift yourself up to your arms, bend your knees, and slide. Did you slide? Did you get stuck? Did you slide too fast and need to grip more?

Everyone is different. This is all about finding your grip and your comfort. If you struggle to lift, I suggest stabilising your grip at face height. Bring one knee up, then the other. You can slightly position the pole between your knees if need be. Then slide down to a kneeling position.

Let's take a look.

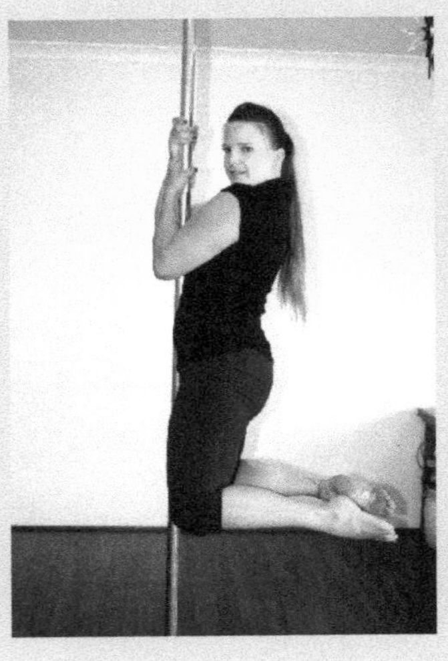

Step 1: Place either arm on the pole at face height (or just above head height). Roll your shoulder back.

Step 2: Place your other hand just below the first.

Step 3: Lift your feet from the floor. Try to keep your arms bent and your hands around face height. This comes with time and practice.

Step 4: Slide to a kneeling position.

Step 5: Now swap hands, placing your other hand on top, and see how the other side goes.

This is just a self-check move, but it helps you get an understanding of your grip. Aim for an even slide, not a release of the arms to hang and then slide. Keep practising! Even use this to practice stopping mid slide if that is what you're training.

Muscles/Areas to Strengthen for the Lift and Slide

- Latissimus dorsi
- Forearm flexors
- Biceps
- Shoulder girdle and scapular stabilisers (trapezius, serratus anterior)
- Rotator cuff (teres minor, infraspinatus)

Muscles to Stretch for the Lift and Slide

- Quads
- Hip flexors

VISUALISATION:
LIFT AND SLIDE

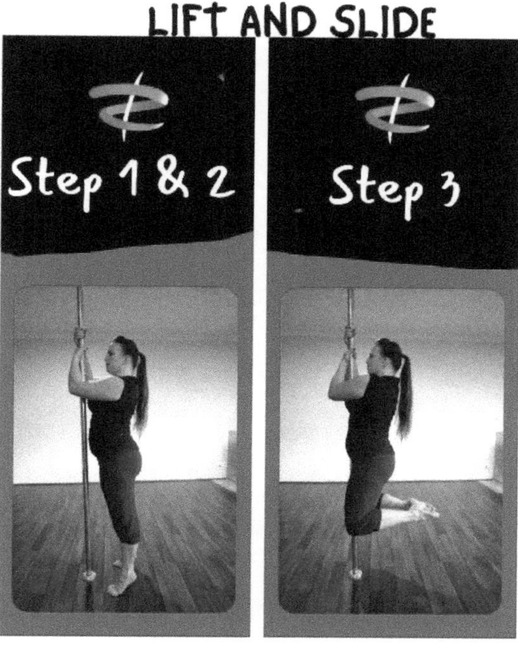

The Pike Spin

We have another new spin to play with, the **pike spin**. This has a technical way and a Lara way. I find that a **technical aerial pike**, very sharp in shape, doesn't flow or spin well and takes a lot more muscle and energy. Plus, it hits that tender point between your knees on the pole. Ouch!

I do more of a crescent moon shape. You can adjust to what suits your body. The pole could be anywhere between the knees, down the calf to the ankles. Basically, with **split grip**, your outside leg comes around straight, tapping the ankle next to the pole. You push off the other foot, and it joins the first on the other side of the pole. As long as your legs are straight next to each other and your feet are together (not crossed), you're good. The **pike spin** is the first step in adjusting your leg alignment and thus changing your centre of gravity slightly while starting in a way you're familiar with.

Here it goes.

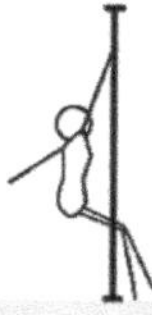

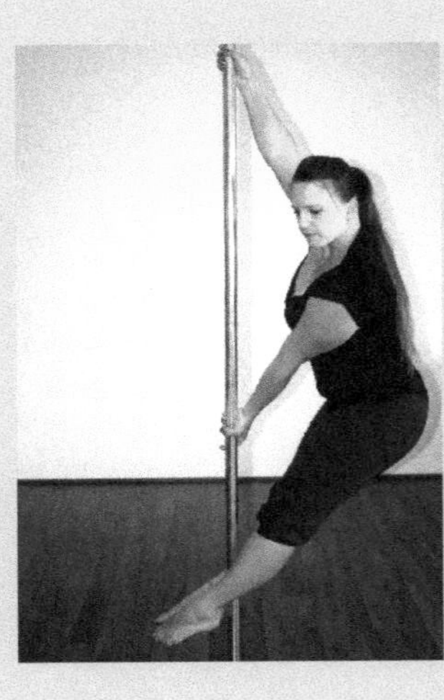

Step 1: Roll your shoulders back, and place your inside hand up, palm facing the direction you're going.

Step 2: Step on your inside leg. Pivot to face the pole.

Step 3: Place your outside hand on the pole with your finger pointing down the pole.

Step 4: Bring your outside leg around in front of the pole, keeping it straight. Pull with your top arm; push with your bottom arm.

Step 5: Use your inside leg to push off the ground, and bring it next to your outside leg.

Step 6: Don't forget to practise both sides, and actively pull with your top arm as you spin.

I find this flows a lot nicer than a strong-angled spin. Remember, it's your body. Find your comfort spot, and flow with it!

If you are still finding split grip to be a struggle, practice one leg at a time, ensure you have safe alignment, activate your grip, bring your toes off the ground. Eventually working to bringing one knee up, then the other knee, then tuck. These will help you solidify your split grip ready for later moves.

Muscles/Areas to Strengthen for the Pike Spin

- Quads
- Adductors
- Shoulder girdle and scapular stabilisers (trapezius, serratus anterior)
- Rotator cuff (teres minor, infraspinatus)
- Forearm flexors
- Elbow stability muscles (if hyper-extensive in the elbows)

Muscles to Stretch for the Pike Spin

- Glutes
- Hamstrings
- Lower back/lumbar

VISUALISATION: PIKE SPIN

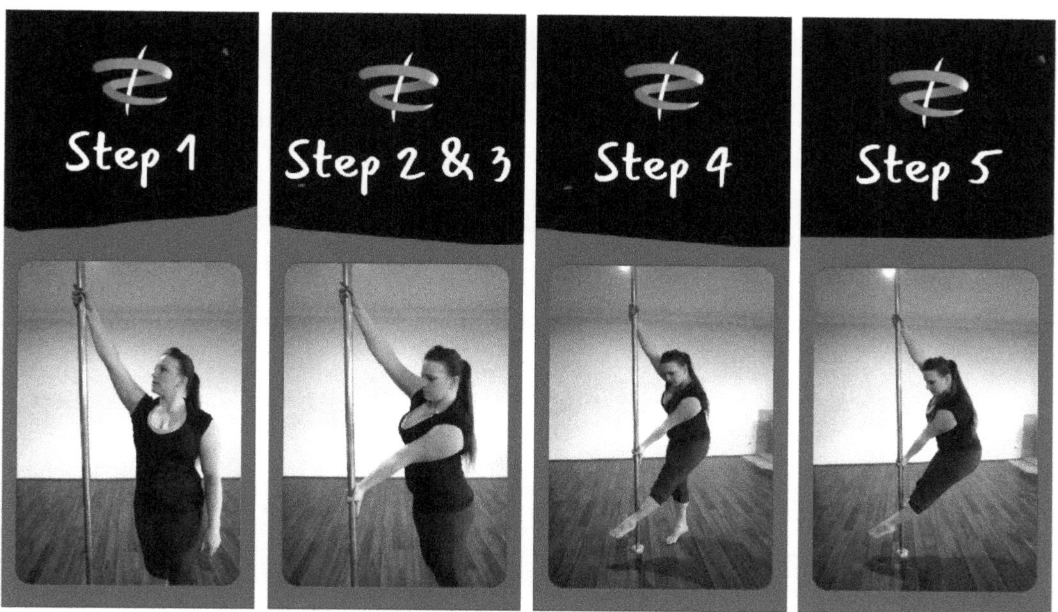

Creating Flow out of our Knee Hook Spins

By this point, you should be pretty solid in your spins, so it's time to look at how to flow or transition out of them nicely and in a manner that protects your joints and creates good habits. Let's have a brief look at a couple of moves we've worked on.

First, the **front-knee hook (forward knees)**. From the spin, what works for me is to put the ball of the foot of the inside leg (the leg around the pole) on the floor. Bring your other leg around in the momentum of the spin, and land both legs together. I find the swoosh brings the leg out wider and gives a different line, and it feels like a lot of fun.

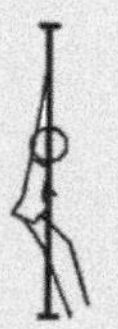

Step 1: Place your inside hand up, palm facing the direction you're going. Roll your shoulders back.

Step 2: Stretch your outside hand across your body, holding on at chest height.

Step 3: Bend your inside leg onto the pole.

Step 4: Stand up on the tippy-toes of your outside leg.

Step 5: Lean forward through your hips, bending the other leg when needed. Let gravity do the work!

Step 6: Put the ball of your inside foot on the floor.

Step 7: Circle your outside leg around the side, and land your feet together. If you can get this leg straight, it's super pretty.

Now let's have a look at the **back-knee hook** (**backward knees**). It's pretty similar. From your spin, this time, your outside foot goes on the floor. Landing on the ball of your foot, pull your hips back to unhook the other leg, bringing that foot through the gap you've made, almost like you're "threading the needle". Keep walking in the same direction. This one is a little more complicated, but once you get the flow, it works. It's also not the only way, but it is one to start you on your journey of experimentation!

Let's take a look.

Step 1: Roll your shoulders back. Place your outside hand up, palm facing the direction you're going (behind you).

Step 2: Wrap your inside hand around the pole at shoulder height.

Step 3: Place your inside foot on its toe in front of the pole. Give it a wiggle to make sure your heel doesn't hit the pole.

Step 4: Transfer your weight onto the ball of your inside foot.

Step 5: Draw a circle behind you with your outside leg.

Step 6: As your calf touches, bend your knees. Spin!

Step 7: Place your outside foot down on the ball of the foot.

Step 8: Pull your hips straight back as you unhook your leg from the pole.

Step 9: Bring that leg through the gap you've created.

Step 10: Keep walking in the same direction (follow the momentum!).

Play with this move until it becomes fluid, and then find your own style and ways to move in and out of moves. You're your own person, so don't think that my way is the only way. It works for me. The special thing about you is that no one else IS you or has your style, so mix it up, and make your style yours!

Conditioning on the Pole: Early Days

Pole Lifts

Pole lifts are great for building foundation strength, and there are so many variations, depending on your level.

Let's start with your hands at head height, shoulders rolled back. Use your hands to pull yourself onto your tippy-toes and lower down again. You aren't lifting your feet off the ground. You're conditioning the muscles that do that, though! Once you're good at that, you can start to slowly control your lower. Controlling the way out is actually training you for getting into the move. Now swap hands. Put your other hand on top, and try again! Always train both sides.

Next options: *(Remember to set your shoulders back and down first!)*

1. Lift to your tippy-toes, then off slightly and down again (do 3 reps on each side; if that's too easy, try 5 on each side).
2. Lift your feet off the ground.
3. Lift your feet off the ground, then lower down.
4. Lift and hold for a count of your choice.
5. Get technical, bringing your hips in front of the pole in your **basic invert grip**, opening a whole new door to lift options! But start with just a basic lift from here, following the above progressions, just with your hips in front.

I've given you a lot of options here, but don't rush them. Spend a number of weeks on each one before moving to the next. You can adjust your counts to increase challenge. But baby steps will get you there. Set a goal of 3 weeks per lift type before moving to the next. That way, you can achieve without feeling disheartened or getting stuck doing the same thing.

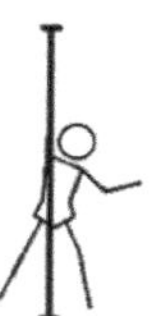

Pole Squats

Next, try **pole squats**. Face the pole with your legs shoulder-width apart. Holding on to the pole, squat with your bottom back. Squat down until your knees are over your ankles and your hips, knees, and shoulders are in line. If your knees go over your toes, this can cause damage, so be aware of your alignment. Now push back through your legs to stand and repeat.

A fun way to step this up is to squat down as you push up to stand. Step one leg to the side, pointing your toes. Then reset and squat down, coming up to point the other toe to the side. And continue.

I enjoy going into a squat, raising up onto the ball of one foot, then the other, then back down to a flat foot on one side and the next foot before standing up again. Then again. Squat, stand up on one toe, other toe, down, down, stand! (When I say toe, I mean the ball of your foot, but thinking 'toe' flows more easily!)

Next up, **pole back slides**. With your back on the pole and your legs in front of the pole, slide down to a squat. Remember, in a squat position, you don't want your knees to go over your toes. You want to move your legs far enough forward that you can squat down to create a tabletop with your thighs. Your knees and ankles should be aligned. You can now push back onto the pole with your upper back to slide back up.

Once you get the hang of this, you can remove stability. Add a new dynamic by kicking one leg out, sliding down to a squat, bringing that foot back to the floor, and pushing back up. Now kick the other leg and repeat. Feel the burn!

Pole Rows

Try **pole rows**. Stand front on with your feet close to the pole, holding the pole with one hand at belly button height. Roll your shoulders back to keep them engaged, lower yourself back/out, and pull back up to the pole, just like if you were using a rowing machine.

Pole Slides

Now for the **pole slide**. Place your hand just above head height, bend at the knees, and slide down onto your knees. While you're still gaining strength to lift yourself off the ground, you can lightly grip the pole between your knees to slide. You may want a mat underneath you to land on while gaining the control to slide.

Have some fun with it

Next, **back-knees spins** and all **basic spins**. However, the **back-knees spin** is less strenuous on the shoulders than many others, as the pole is more sideways.

Try pole moves, even dance ones. **False step-arounds** provide opportunities to gain strength. Hip circles and squatting down and up are fun and strengthening. Don't get stuck in all the conditioning. Pick moves that are specific to your skills, or practise your moves. Put some music on, and find your flow!

I like to spend 10 minutes training lots of moves, working more muscles than I would if I focused on just a couple of muscle groups. But this depends on your pole goals and what you plan on achieving. Controlling your way out of moves is one of the best ways to get control for going into them, so look at your dismounts, and make them neat and controlled.

Eventually, you can move on to **tabletop lifts**, **pole tucks**, and other fun things!

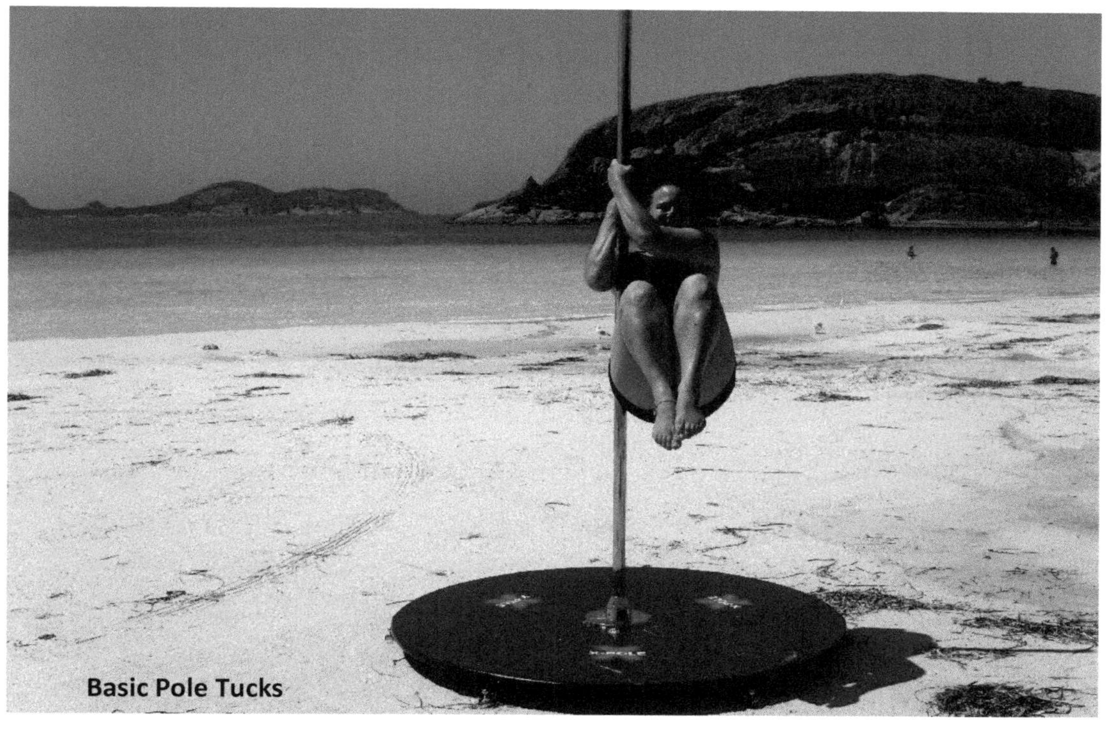

Basic Pole Tucks

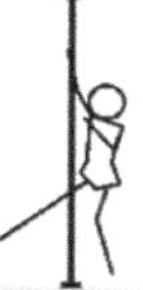

Getting Technical: What You've Learnt So Far

Let's recap what you've done so far. Now it's all making sense. Flow is starting to come, so before you create bad habits, let's get technical and add more depth (or lift) to your moves.

Use your Wings!

The most important floaty move is using your wings. Imagine you have a set of wings just below the back of your shoulder blades. As you spin, try to pull down on your wings, and use them to give you lift. You'll notice that you feel like you're flying. This technique also adds a lot more lift to your moves. This makes you use the bigger muscles of your back to lift instead of the smaller arm muscles, and it makes you align and actively control your grip.

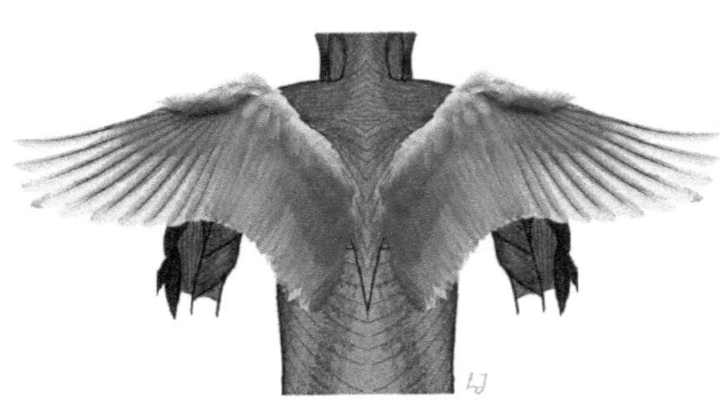

In the circus aerial world, your wings have a lot to do with the lower part of your trapezius muscle (along with your serratus anterior and rotator cuff muscles). The lower trapezius maintains the shoulder blade on the trunk, so it sits nicely and doesn't hang out at funny angles. Yes, there are lots of other little muscles at work as well, but using the lower trapezius muscle, it effectively lifts the body to the shoulder blade. This is what gives you the floaty feeling as you spin. When used effectively, the spin feels completely different; the hanging and heaviness are gone! It's ironic that the kite-looking muscle is the one that makes you fly.

Many moves don't work if you aren't actively using your grip. Just hanging from your arm doesn't cut it. You'll also notice that if you're hanging from your top arm instead of actively pulling with it, the forearm of your bottom arm will start to ache. Also, if you are not activating the right muscles, or setting your grip incorrectly, you will increase tension in your neck, ensure your neck and shoulders are relaxed.

Want to work more on shoulder stability? Neola Wilby, the pole PT, uses fit balls to help, as it can be tricky to stabilise muscles surrounding big joints like your shoulders and hips. Core and shoulder stability are the foundation of all pole movements. All those different twists and flows constantly move through these areas, so they're important to work on. Eventually, you'll get strong enough to progress to more advanced styles and moves.

Safety in training

Safety in training is a massive thing. Seeing so many unsafe practices is the reason I wrote this book. We want to have fun, enjoy this magical sport, and stay injury-free. A lot of safety has to do with listening to your body. How often should you train? How long should you train for? How intensely should you train? These things are different for everyone.

Tracking these also helps you work out your rhythm and body, did you have enough sleep, are you already fatigued prior to training. How different do you feel before, and after training, how quickly did you fatigue? Making note of how you are feeling allows you to really notice what your body puts in and needs during each training session, and the appropriate intensity of that training session. Remember pain is not normal, please don't "push through the pain" instead get it professionally looked into to find out why there is pain in the first place.

It's a good idea to sketch out a plan – weekly, monthly, seasonally, leading up to a performance, or whatever suits your busy life! It isn't just about training on the pole. You want to look at cross-training, strength training, and rest days too. Want to go gung-ho? Train on the pole 3 to 5 times a week, but add in some cardio 2 to 3 days a week, giving your shoulders a rest.

To keep things even, you can do some strength training 2 to 3 days a week, but remember to also look at muscles other than those you train on the pole, and balance yourself out. Make sure to factor in rest days. Ensure that you always warm up and cool down before and after training sessions.

The book *Applied Anatomy of Aerial Arts* by Emily Scherb, DPT has a great rundown of injuries in aerials and understanding what they are and how they feel.[8]

Hand Positioning

Hand positioning makes sense when you get it. At the beginning, though, you have to fight the urge to lower your top arm to lift onto the pole. It seems that the brain's natural inclination is to think 'up' to get your feet off the floor. You'll really feel like you need to lift up! On the other hand, some people feel the need to put their hand so height their arm is almost handing out of their shoulder.

With spinning, this isn't the case. You should position your hands where they naturally want to sit on the pole, keeping your arms straight and your shoulders rolled back and activated. If you feel your shoulders pushing back strangely, readjust your hand height. Once your hands are correctly positioned, you'll find it easier to create your pull/push scenario.

Keep your bottom hand in mind. If you put it lower in your **basic grip** and create an **extended basic grip**, you'll be putting more pressure on your wrist. If you're unable to reach across your chest, it's safer to go with a higher (more of a baseball) grip than a lower one. Just as with the **split grip**, pointing your finger down the pole aligns straight pressure down your arm into the pole. A twist in your wrist here isn't a strong position and can cause weakness and damage. Think of placing the dip in your bottom hand on the pole with your finger facing down. If your finger wraps, your wrist twists.

Does your wrist Wrap?

Think about your top hand. Does your wrist wrap? This may mean you're not actively using your top arm and are hanging out of it more than if you lifted through your shoulder blades. The first thing to try is focusing on actively pulling with your top arm. You'll notice that wrist strength develops with time, and this is also a factor. You want your wrist to maintain alignment in your arm. That active pulling will help here.

If you're still struggling, grab a sweatband or a scrunchie, and pop it around your wrist. This will decrease the friction on your wrist while you work on correcting technique and strengthening your wrist. Be aware that if you are persistent and don't fix the problem, friction burn can happen.

Grip

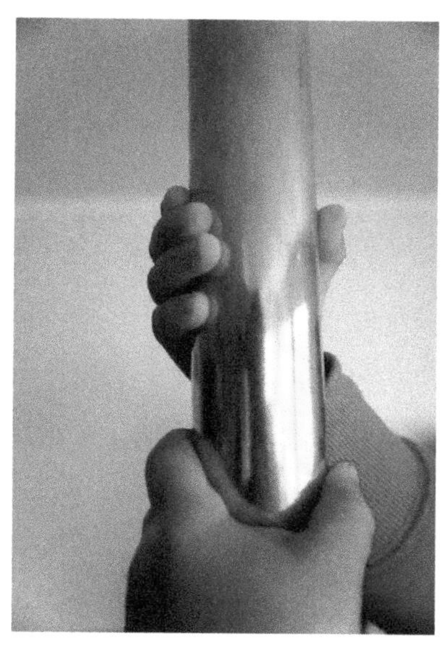

So, we have worked out all grips on the pole work on a push/pull scenario. One arm is pulling, the other arm or limb, has an element of push onto the pole. We have also learnt to actively ensure we are pulling with our top arm, always rolling back our shoulders to not hang out of the socket. Remember, if you experience a pain in your forearm in split grip, it may mean that you are not actively pulling with your top arm, and thus, overloading the bottom. However, if this is not the case, seek advice from a healthcare professional.

We just re-capped wrists wrapping during spins; but it is also worth being aware of the angle of which your hand is wrapping around the pole for static holds. Is your arm going straight to your wrist and then the pole? Or are you wrapping your hand around the pole a little? This wrap, many people do it, it means that you sometimes move when you don't want to. If you are holding your weight stably in a wrapped hand, your body will move, to align with the wrist again and maintain a straight line. So, as you progress your journey, if you find you are moving around the pole, when you don't feel as if you should, check your alignment. Have you created straight lines onto the pole, or is your body moving to create that straight line?

Also remember to do your hand and finger warm ups, get your hands ready to look after you. If you still find grip a struggle, try different width poles, find what suits your body.

Dynamic Levels

Dynamic levels are amazing. Creating levels in your routine is so important, not only for aesthetics but also for muscle balance and fatigue. Things look prettier and retain interest for longer if they aren't all at the same level. Breaking up moves with different types of moves – going up the pole or floorwork, in the case of a spin routine – also gives your muscles a chance to rest before continuing. Getting the hang of some

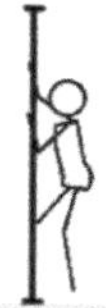

floorwork helps for slippery or fatiguing days so that you can flow through and continue on like nothing is wrong instead of being completely stumped.

Transitioning in and out of moves

Getting in and out of a move should be considered part of the move. That way, if you have a bail-out day, your body and mind won't think, 'Okay, I'm there; let go now!' The move won't be finished. Training from the beginning to get in and out of moves nicely isn't just a good habit because it looks pretty; it's imperative for the safety of your muscles. Dropping and plonking out of moves is dangerous. If you are fatigued and that's what you do, you're more likely to injure yourself. If all your body knows is to get in and out of things nicely, even on a bad day, that's what will be natural, and no one will know it's a bad day!

Practise different transitions and different ways in and out of moves, and remember, the move isn't finished until you land it nicely. Land and strike a pose if you like!

Again, actively pulling in your grips is so important. Use your wings, and fly!

Straight Lines

Creating a straight line with your body when looking at directional force really helps you feel secure. Alignment and lines in your body assist you to utilise the correct muscles, and to not feel as if you are wobbly or unstable. Create momentum by pulling with your top arm and pushing your leg away from you. This line feels stable, all your muscles are activated to hold the line. Instead of feeling wishy-washy and not feeling strong in your positions. Taking photos and videos helps you to look at the lines your body creates and you can then relate them to how you felt and look at what works for you.

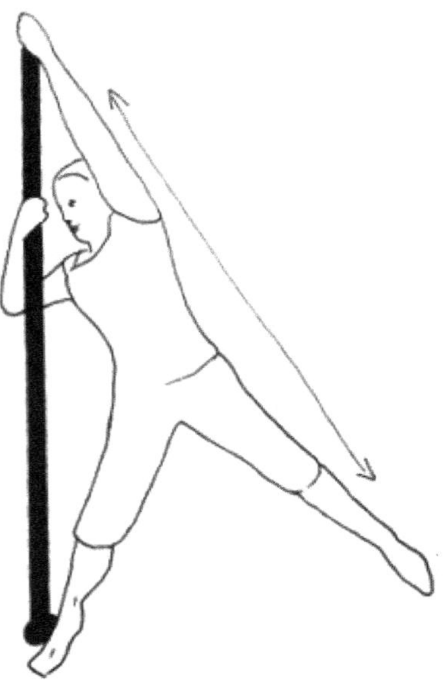

Learning About the Pelvic Floor

There is a forgotten muscle that, unless you've had a baby or your partner has had one, you may not know exists. But it is such an integral muscle. Sure, it helps you go to the toilet. But it does so much more than that.

Think of your pelvic floor like a boat that you sit on. Your hips are joined to it. Your back is joined to it. And it joins where your abs connect. It literally cups your torso. This boat is more of a ship; it has lots of masts coming off it. So what?

Do you get lower-back aches? There's a chance it could be your pelvic floor not activating to hold everything up. Let's go back to the boat analogy. Boats have masts. If the boat wasn't sturdy, would the masts stand strong? No! If your pelvic floor isn't sturdy, it affects your whole torso. Muscles start making up for other muscles that aren't doing their job. One bit gets tight and sore, and the other relaxes, causing all sorts of chaos, all because of a forgotten muscle! Your pelvic floor affects your hips, and if your hips are out, so are your shoulders. The problem works its way up your body.

Not forgotten your pelvic floor? Sweet! But remember, it does need to be released too. Don't try to hold it all day every day!

How can you find your pelvic floor without going to the toilet and stopping yourself from weeing? Sit on the floor cross-legged. Most of the muscles touching the floor underneath you are your pelvic floor. Think of squeezing upwards right in the middle. No, not squeezing your bottom. Your glutes will make you relax your pelvic floor. Squeeze that section right in front of your bottom; draw it up! Confusing, right?

Okay, girls. Imagine there is a peanut underneath you that you want to pick up with your vagina. (Please don't actually pick anything up with your vagina; hygiene!) Did that help?

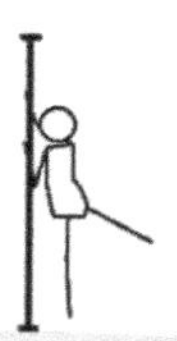

Boys, your pelvic floor muscles can also weaken with age, and they totally exist as a hammock from the tail bone to the pubic bone. Imagine your penis is a straw. Pretend, using your internal muscles, to draw up through that straw (again, hygiene; please don't try to drink through your newfound phallic straw). Is that concept working for you? How about walking into a cold lake and feeling your testicles draw up towards you? That's probably a more relatable feeling. Meet your pelvic floor.

There are all sorts of things you can do to strengthen these muscles, but this isn't my area of expertise. The main thing is to be aware of them. They're an important part of maintaining posture and correct body alignment.

Please note: some people are overactive, while others are underactive in their pelvic floor. Creating your own pelvic floor exercise routine, however good your intentions, can backfire. Being aware of your pelvic floor's existence in pole is generally enough. If you feel the need or have queries and questions, talk to a professional in the field.

Starting to Lift

I'm going to start here with the move that takes up more energy, just so that it isn't so fatiguing at the end of training. However, I do recommend practising a few things you know already to re-orientate yourself with the pole after your warm-up.

The Fireman to Pole Stand

This looks like a daunting move, but it isn't really. Meet the **fireman-to-pole stand**. This takes you back to the first **fireman** you learnt, the **basic spin grip**, with your legs in a position where all of the skin of the calf was in contact with the pole. It's important here that the pole stays between your knees, as that helps you get higher up the pole, like from your knee to your crotch. If the pole is mid-thigh, there isn't much space between the pole and the crotch, so you won't get up high or feel as if you're achieving.

VISUALISATION: POLE SQUAT

Step 1 & 2

Step 3

Let's practise.

Hold the pole at chest height. Squat down, feet on either side of the pole, pole between your knees. Now squeeze (on the squishy part). Bring your hips up at 45 degrees to the pole, keeping your torso straight and looking at the pole. (Shoot your torso up like a rocket ship!) That's the movement you want to do on the pole.

When spinning, if you bring your hips straight to the pole, your knees will just slide down, so you need to think 'up'. I think so much 'up' that after my hips go up, I move my bottom hand up too. But this is just helping my mental cue of 'up-ness'.

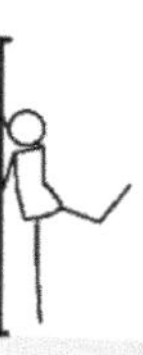

A lot of people try to look up and lead with their chest in their lift. This deactivates the core muscles. Try something for me. Lie on the ground, and do a sit up. Now look up above your head (behind you), and try to do a sit-up. See how much harder that is? You want to keep your core activated and straight, so keep your torso straight. And look at the pole or your hands the whole time.

Think of it like rock climbing. If a rock climber used their hands to climb, they would fatigue quickly. Use your bigger muscles: your legs! Stand up on your legs instead of lifting up with your hands. Squeeze the pole at the same time. Again, try it from the ground if you need to help your body know what to do before adding the elements of height and spin.

Time to look at the spin, starting with your **basic fireman spin**.

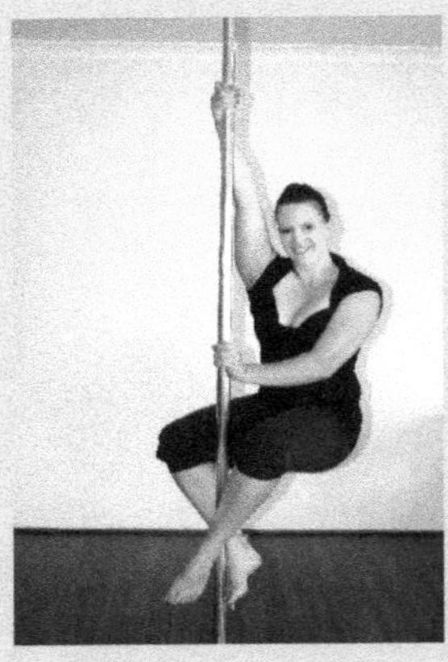

Step 1: Place your inside hand up on the pole, palm facing the direction you're going. Roll your shoulders back.

Step 2: Stretch your outside hand across your body, holding on at chest height.

Step 3: Step on your inside leg to bring your outside leg in front of the pole (knee on one side, ankle on the other), all of the skin of your calf on the pole.

Step 4: Tap your other leg to the back of the pole (knee on one side, ankle on the other so that one knee is on each side of the pole). Again, place as much skin as you can get on the pole.

Now let's change it up. Remember what we broke down. From the start of this spin, squeeze your knees. Hips up; hands up. Ready?

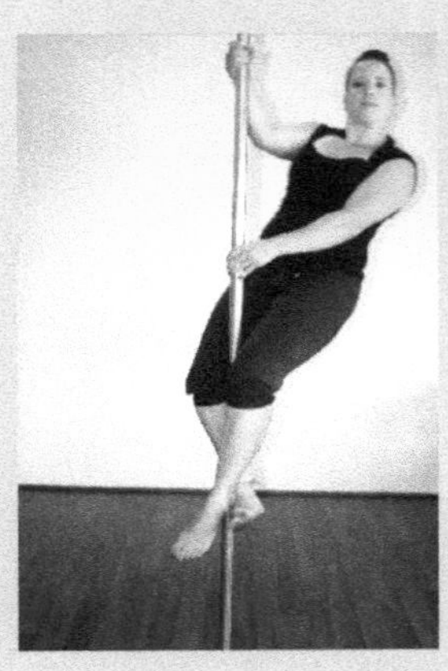

Step 1: Place your inside hand up, palm facing the direction you're going. Roll your shoulder back.

Step 2: Stretch your outside hand across your body, holding on at chest height.

Step 3: Step on your inside leg to bring your outside leg in front of the pole (knee on one side, ankle on the other). Rest all of the skin of your calf on the pole.

Step 4: Tap your other leg to the back of the pole (knee on one side, ankle on the other so that one knee is on each side of the pole). Again, put as much skin as you can get on the pole.

Step 5: Start to spin.

Step 6: Squeeze your legs together on the pole.

Step 7: Bring your hips up 45 degrees to stand.

Step 8: Optional- bring your bottom hand up to chest height.

Sweet! How do you feel after that? It can be exhausting. It uses different movements and muscles from anything you've done so far. But it feels amazing to finally get it. It's like the next step has been unlocked!

This one on a spinning pole really spins, so be prepared. This is the reason for my slight lean back in the photo; I was trying to slow the spin!

This move is a whole new step, a whole new strength and movement in your pole journey. Take a look at the QR code to get a better understanding of how it works. Just remember, hips up! Not "to" the pole, bringing them "to" the pole means your legs will slide down. Bringing them up, gives you the height, allowing your legs to maintain their grip.

VISUALISATION: FIREMAN TO POLE STAND

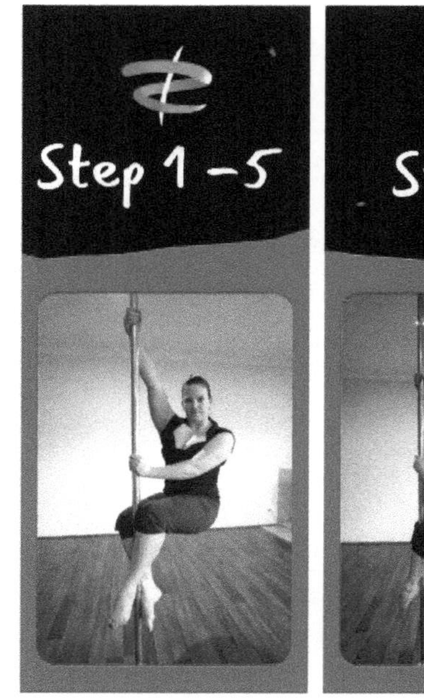

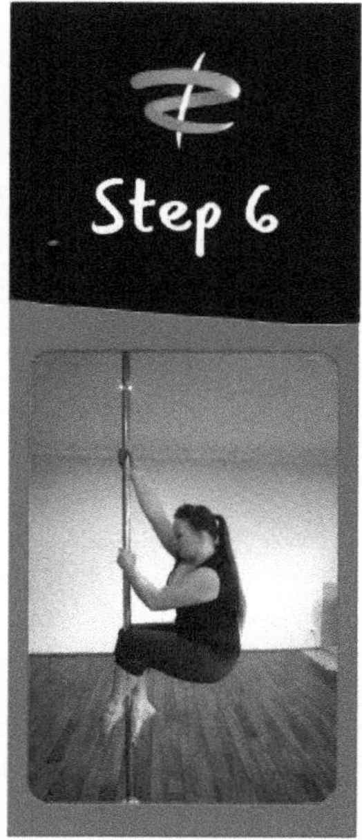

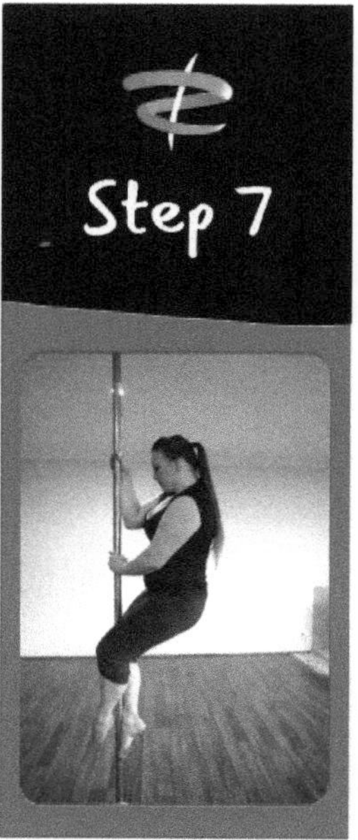

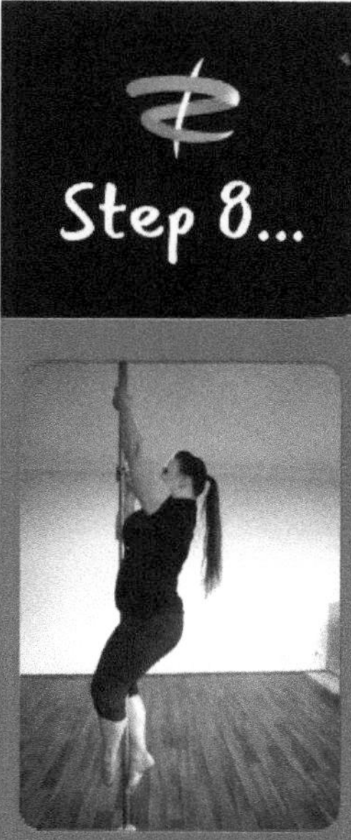

Muscles/Areas to Strengthen for the Fireman-to-Pole Stand

- Same as **basic fireman spin:**
    - Hip flexors
    - Shoulder girdle and scapular stabilisers (trapezius, serratus anterior)
    - Rotator cuff (teres minor, infraspinatus)
    - Core (abs, back, and pelvic floor)
- Quads

Muscles to Stretch for the Fireman-to-Pole Stand

- Same as **basic fireman spin:**
    - Glutes
    - Hamstrings
    - Triceps
    - Latissimus dorsi
    - Pectorals

The Straddle Spin

The **straddle spin (also known as boomerang)** is the next step. I really like this spin. It's the start of changing your body shape around the pole, removing your legs to properly rely on the push/pull of your **split grip**.

Think of sitting down on the floor in a **straddle stretch**, except you're up on the pole, spinning. The height of your legs on this one comes with time. Get used to the flow of the move before looking at activating your quads and core to lift your legs up more. You want to keep your torso upright. You aren't leaning into this move or sticking your bottom out. You're rolling your shoulders back to pull with your top hand and push with your bottom hand.

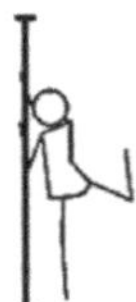

If **split grip** isn't working for you, you can also do your **straddle spin** in **forearm grip**, as you can really pull back through your shoulder and still tuck your pelvis under to get the straddle. It does take some practice to avoid letting your forearm slide off the pole, though.

Get into your **split grip**, then place your legs in position (don't rush it and try to do it all at once). Your outside leg comes up nice and straight and bring it around until it is almost at the pole. Now shift focus to the other leg. Push through the ball of your foot on your inside leg to lift it, keeping it straight. This push gives momentum for the spin.

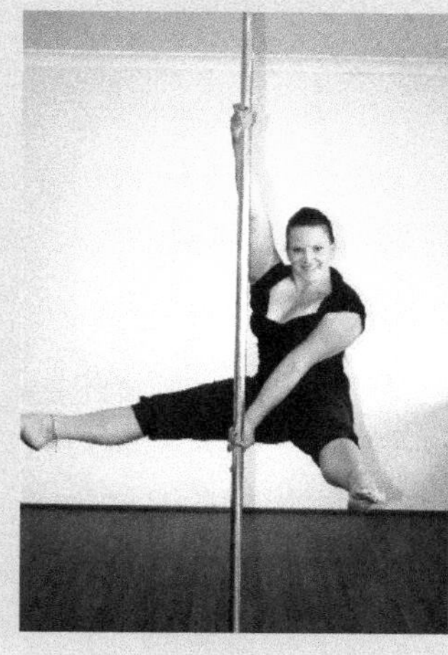

Step 1: Roll your shoulders back. Place your inside hand up, palm facing the direction you're going.

Step 2: Step on your inside leg. Pivot to face the pole.

Step 3: Place your outside hand on the pole with your finger pointing down the pole.

Step 4: Bring your outside leg up and around, stopping before you get to the pole. Pull with your top arm; push with your bottom arm.

Step 5: Push off your inside leg as you bring it up to spin.

Don't be afraid to start with your toes pointing down. Baby steps! Get used to the motion. Straddle position; legs straight. Once it flows, look at lifting your legs higher.

Your straddle doesn't need a massive amount of flexibility. Move within your comfort range. As you progress through your pole journey, you'll come across more flexible moves.

Something to keep in mind is to only use a maximum of 85% of your flexibility or movement ability to achieve these moves. This allows you a slim margin for error. If you use 100% of your movement ability and get sweaty and slip, you're in trouble! This also allows you to feel more comfortable and in control of the move than if you pushed it to its limits. This is a tip to keep in mind, as everyone thinks flexible thoughts when doing their **straddle spin**, but you should be moving in your own personal range of motion here. The risks are much lower!

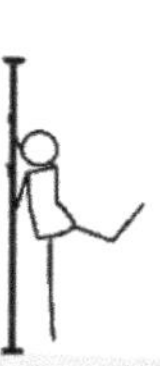

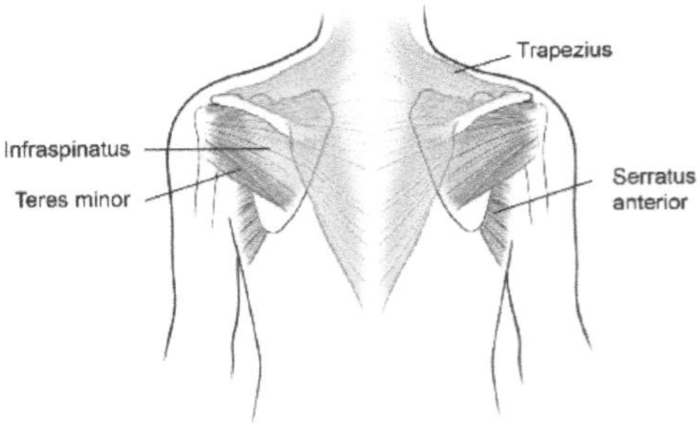

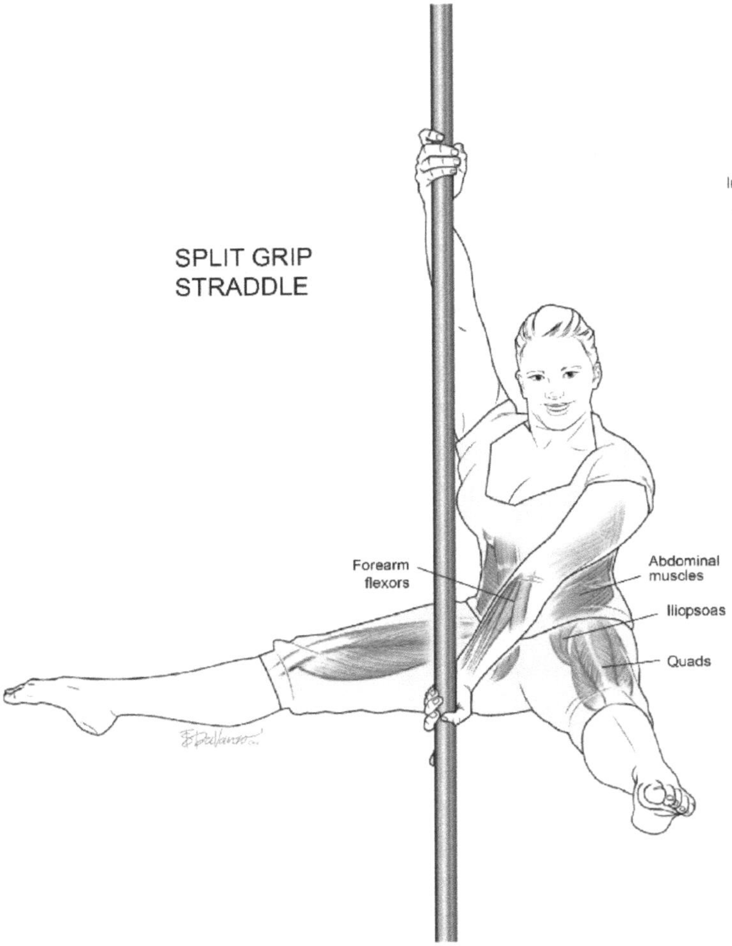

Muscles/Areas to Strengthen for the Straddle Spin

- Hip flexors
- Abdominals
- Shoulder girdle and scapular stabilisers (trapezius, serratus anterior)
- Rotator cuff (teres minor, infraspinatus)
- Forearm flexors
- Elbow stability muscles (if hyper-extensive in the elbows)

Muscles to Stretch for the Straddle Spin

- Glutes
- Hamstrings
- Lower back/lumbar

VISUALISATION: STRADDLE SPIN

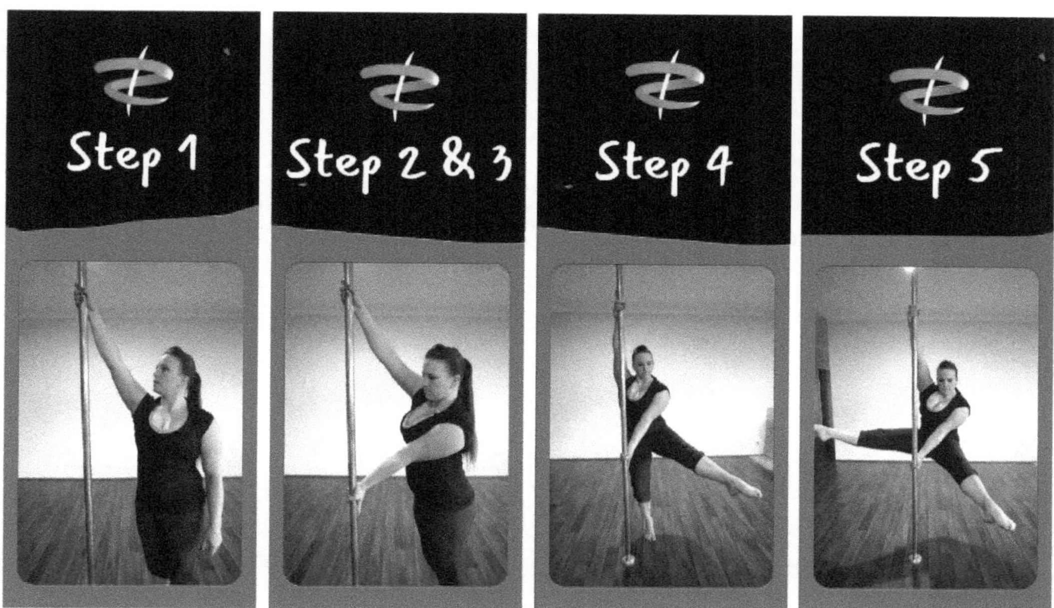

Backward Spiral Spin

From here, you should have enough control to start playing with leg variations from spins you've learnt. One of those is the **backward spiral**. The hardest part of this move is telling your body not to do what it knows how to do. This is one of the reasons why it's good to mix it up early before you get stuck in habits. It gives you more fluidity to play.

The **backward spiral** starts off just like the **back-knee hook**. You have your **reverse spin grip**. This one is a bit less complicated with the legs, though. You're going to circle your outside leg like in the **backward-knee hook** but with a bit more lift to try and make it flatter.

The other (inside) leg lifts up, toe to knee. The toe of your inside foot should point to the knee of your outside leg. Sit it on the ground. Your hip is next to the pole, and your outside leg is bent out to the side, the foot facing behind you. Your inside knee is bent forward, pointing your toe to your outside knee. This is the position you're after on the pole. It requires a fair bit of oblique crunch (and glute med) to get the flat effect.

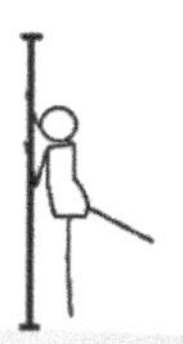

This is a fantastic move to spin all the way to the floor, as you can then self-check without a mirror. Which part of your body lands first? Your knees? Lift more with your side (oblique). What position are your legs in when they land? Are they making the right shape? Generally, your thigh touches the pole in this spin. If you get extra momentum, though, it may get a bit airborne. Just try to not swing out into the move, or you'll swing back onto the pole! Ouch.

Let's do it.

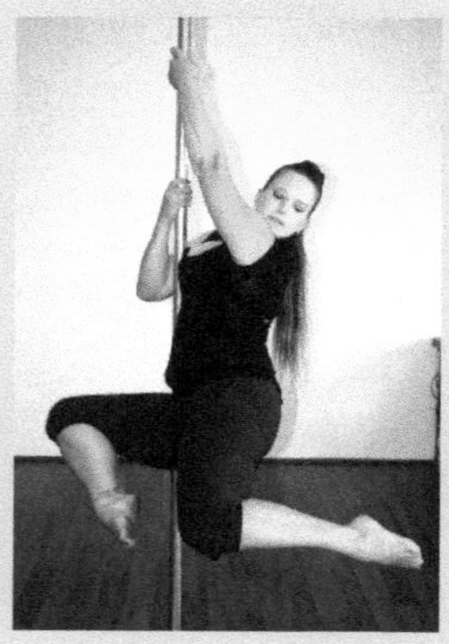

Step 1: Roll your shoulder back. Place your outside hand up, palm facing the direction you're going (behind you).

Step 2: Wrap your inside hand around the pole at shoulder height.

Step 3: Draw a circle going behind you with your outside leg.

Step 4: Lift your inside toe to your knee. Spin!

Remember to try both sides and take it to the floor. Have a look. How did you land? What shape? Where are your legs? Think about this, and try again until you create a shape you like.

Muscles/Areas to Strengthen for the Backward Spiral

- Gluteus medius
- Abductors
- Trunk (abs, obliques)
- Shoulder girdle and scapular stabilisers (trapezius, serratus anterior)
- Rotator cuff (teres minor, infraspinatus)

Muscles to Stretch for the Backward Spiral

- Hip flexors
- Side (obliques)
- Hip adductors

Remember to look at your transitions!

Practise these moves for a couple of weeks, then look at coming out of them nicely.

VISUALISATION: BACKWARDS SPIRAL

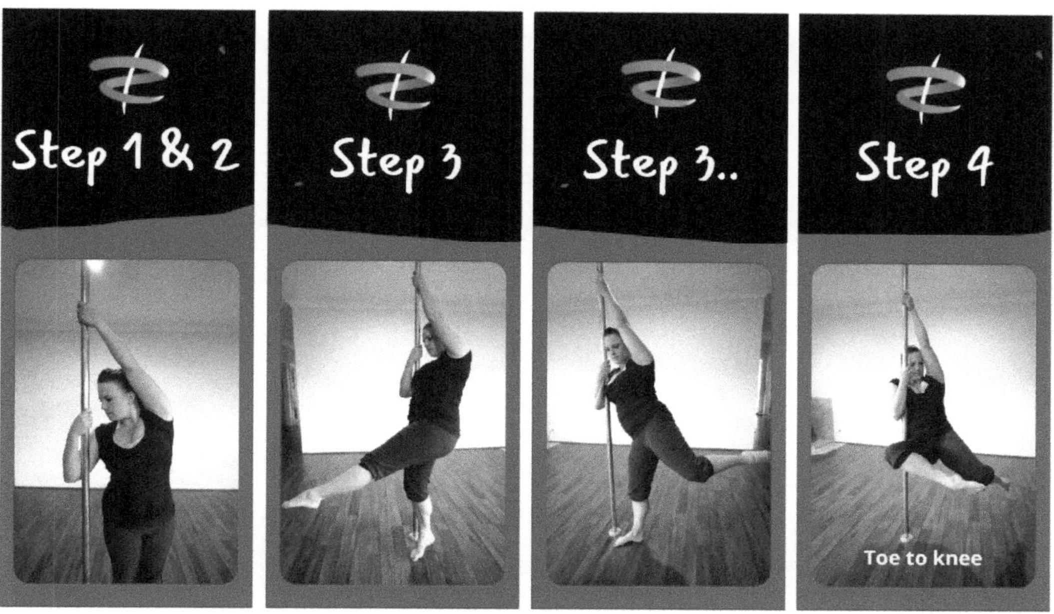

Some moves have fun little tricks you can use to smooth them out. For example, stepping out of your **straddle spin**. Get comfortable with the spin first, then look at how to place your legs down to get out of this move. It's a lot easier in the **straddle spin** to plonk your legs down, which isn't amazing for your joints. To step out of this spin, try bending your back leg (the one that's trailing behind you). When you bend this leg mid-spin, your body has a slight turn, allowing your legs to come together more easily. Here, bring your bent leg to your leading front leg, and walk out of the move. Place whichever leg is natural for you down first.

With the backwards spiral, I generally train it to the ground, not only for extra conditioning, but as I don't have a mirror to see my leg placement. However, you can't just leave it at that. Find unique and elegant or flowing ways to get up from the ground. What leg flairs or floor work can you add in after landing the spin? Eventually, training ways to get out of the move without coming to the ground but maintaining the flow and momentum that the spin has created.

Finishing Moves

I've already covered this, I know. But from a safety perspective, it's worth covering again. When training any move, even those that are upside down on the pole, you shouldn't consider it finished until you're on the ground, 2 feet next to each other and no weight-bearing in your arms.

Yes, I'm quite specific here. No staggered sloppy-footed landing. Place your feet nicely! Your feet and arms could be placed and posed. That's perfectly fine. But if you're not looking for a particular shape, work out how to land, bringing your feet together and no longer holding your weight on the pole.

This is even something with inverts. You're not done when you're in the move (upside down). You're not done when you can touch the floor. The move is finished when you're grounded on the floor safely (and prettily, of course!). Confused?! Basically, if you still have the need to grip the pole with your hands or legs, you are not finished the move (in saying that, when inverted, please use all grip points necessary). If you have controlled your descent and have landed in a grounded manner, you won't need to support your body with the pole, then you have finished the move. Where you then place your limbs for following transitions is your choice.

One of my funny focuses is the floating hand. During moves where your hand is not in use, even walks, your hand must have a purpose. Putting it on your hip is fine. Otherwise, point it, trace the side of your body, wave it around like you're in the 1960s – purposefully. As long as the floating hand has a job! If it doesn't, it tends to detract from the move, and some people's eyes will wander to that hand, anticipating what's going to happen next. Create lines and purpose, and don't let your hand float. Even after a move, where have you placed your hands? Or your feet? They must have a purposeful position and pose, or they take away from everything else.

The same goes for pointed toes. If your feet are flexed, it should be purposeful. Otherwise, finish the line you're creating down your leg to your toes. Lines and angles are beautiful, and those lines and angles are what will make you stand out as you perform. And finish your moves!

Fatiguing? Give that move a rest. Yes, repetition helps you learn. However, your brain-body (or neuromotor) pathways can also fatigue. This explains those frustrating moments when you don't feel tired but what you're practising is going downhill the more you do it. If you keep practising your sloppy, fatigued technique, that's what your neuromotor pathways will start to remember, thus making bad technique your default. Give your nervous system a rest, and go back to that move another day when your body is fresh to practise good technique and finish it nicely.

The pole physio has some great tips to help you notice when you hit this rest point so that you can keep yourself safe and train to the best of your ability.

Pointing Your Toes

Note: we're talking about lots of small bones, tendons, and muscles, so please don't be rough! You don't want to strain or overexert your feet. (Strangely enough, I am being serious here!)

How do you know you're not doing it properly?

Are you engaging your toes only? You need to engage your whole foot to the point where you can feel your point in your calf muscle. Your calf muscle is at the back of your leg, in the lower half or under the knee, the part that looks AMAZING in high heels.

Are you pushing through your heel? Again, your whole foot needs to be activated.

Think about making your body longer. Extend your feet. Can you make your leg look longer by sitting down and extending your feet?

You really have to break each movement down, which can be quite tedious. Flex your foot, engage the ankle and the ball of the foot, and push through the ball of the foot, making it reach away from your body as far as possible. Now start to point your toes down to feel your arch muscles activate. Voila! Pointed toes! It's not passive, is it? You have to work for it, but it gets easier with practice.

Exercises You Can Do

- Floorwork. Bow and arrow. Not only can you trace your toes down your leg from knee to toe and make it look ridiculously sensual as you lower that leg and trace it back again; it's conditioning too! Pull your belly button to the ground, and your core will go berserk. The lower you let your legs go, the more intense it will become. This also works your glutes and promotes stability. Keep your muscles engaged, and remember, slow is sensual, so don't rush! If you're struggling, start with your legs higher, tracing your toe down your leg a little bit. Slowly trace further and further, then lower your legs more and more.

Imagine you're wearing French silk stockings that you just have to touch and caress with your toe.

- Technical foot biomechanics movements. You're still on your back, and your legs are straight up to the roof. Now break down the little foot things. Flex your foot so it's flat like you're standing on a ceiling. Now, keeping your toes pointing to the wall, bend your ankle so the rest of your foot points to the roof. Think of it as pushing through the ball of your foot. This has a name: demi-pointe. Now point your toes to the roof and reverse it. Keep your toes pointing to the ceiling, and flex your foot. Then release your toes to point to the wall again. Repeat.
- Ankle circles. One way, then the other. Do it until you can really feel it working your muscles.
- Resistance band wonderment. Sitting on the floor, legs out in front of you, pop a resistance band around the ball of your foot. Keeping your toes to the roof, drive the ball of your foot to a point, and point your toes, again breaking down each movement. Release and repeat. Think of keeping your toes long; don't scrunch! Feel free to play with the length of your band to make it easier or harder.
- Stretch your foot. Go up onto your toes and back down. Standing toe rises are awesome. You can also pop the tops of your toes on the ground and stretch your foot forward. Stretching can be done in steps without putting weight on the foot. Do one foot at a time. Bring one foot slightly forward (this helps with balance). Bring it up onto the ball of the foot, then up onto the toe, then back to the ball of the foot, and then flat next to you. You've just moved through the motions of each joint in your foot. Now transfer weight, and repeat on the other side. Remember, you're not weighting the foot. You're just moving and bringing it back to centre.
- Massage balls. They're quite amazing. While supporting yourself on something, get a soft, squishy massage ball, and roll it around the underside of your foot. You can even rest it under your heel and stand on it if you have a ball that's soft and sturdy enough. It's quite a nice release, and it gets everything flowing and moving in your foot.

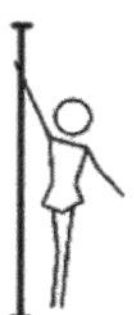

- Calf raises. To do these, lift onto the balls of your feet. It's also good practice to do the reverse of every movement, so lowering your heel over a step (holding on to something so you don't fall back) is also a good idea.
- Muscle activation. Look at muscle groups you don't normally use, like those around the arch of the foot. Can you focus entirely on activating them? It's tricky at first. Think of engaging your arch to scrunch your foot together without any part of your foot leaving the ground. Some people find it easier to have a coin under the ball of the foot so they can visualise pushing it back. Others like to do this but use a pen under the arch, imagining lifting the foot away from the pen while pushing on the coin. Be aware that without being warmed up, pushing your arch too far can cause a cramp.

If you point too hard too quickly, especially if you're not used to it, you will get cramps! Now what?

Use a tennis ball or a small foam roller. Roll lightly over the cramped area and the area around it. Tennis balls are great, as you can go more circular, and the muscles soon begin to ease. Don't just focus on the cramping muscles; massage all around them too! If you have a soft, spiky massage ball, you can also try that.

Alternatively, add warmth using a hot water bottle or a heat pad/pack, or just soak in warm water.

Hydrate. You should do this all the time anyway, but make sure you hydrate if you're cramping.

Your skin grips differently depending on your muscles. If the muscles underneath are actively engaged, grip becomes easier.

Pointing your toes is like a foundation. If your feet are stronger, your body weight is dispersed better, and your foundation is stronger. Going up the line, if your feet are aligned, the rest of your body should be aligned and functioning too. So many people have neck or other issues that come from their feet! This may not be your case, but it is an example of how important a good foundation is and how incorrect alignment can travel through the body.

Learning Basic Floorwork

The world of floorwork is massive and amazing. Here are some moves that you don't need kneepads or shoes for. Shoes make toe slides amazing and dramatic; kneepads help if you're doing a fair bit of work. But let's have a look at a few more resting floorwork options. These can help you bring down the energy levels (or at least your personal energy output) but still finish a routine if you start to get too slippery or tired.

You've already had a look at the **windmill**, but let's recap while you're on the floor.

Step 1: Kick across your body.

Step 2: Use your foot to circle up to the roof as you bring your second leg out to the side.

Step 3: Bring your first leg out to your side as the following foot points to the roof, then to the side.

Step 4: Follow the momentum, and roll onto your belly.

There's a whole range of things you can do on your back or propped up on your elbows. Eventually, when you get candlestick on the floor, you can play with these there. That will give you the opportunity to add some dynamic levels to your floorwork as well. Note: candlestick is advanced floorwork, as your body positioning requires more control and you need to ensure your weight is distributed as to not put pressure on your head or neck. Not sure what candlestick is? Picture your toes pointed up to the roof, as your hands support your hips in the air. I will not go more in-depth than that, as it is not something you should try without proper tuition.

The world of low pole and floorwork is a whole other kettle of fish, so let's look at some basics.

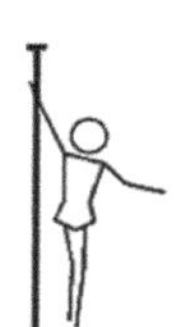

Little Kicks

Try **little kicks**. Lying on your back (or elbows/position of choice), bring your legs straight up, toes pointed to the roof. Keeping your knees together, bring one foot at a time, bending at the knee, down to point towards the ground and back up again. Now do **little kicks** back and forth; point your toe to the floor, then point toe to roof as the other foot does the opposite.

The speed of any of these moves is up to you, your style, and the music. Don't be afraid to make floor moves slow and dramatic. Sometimes, fast can look messy and panicked unless purposefully placed.

Tear Drops

From here, you can also look at **teardrops**, which also start with your legs together, your toes pointing to the roof. There are single and double-leg versions of this. With **double-leg teardrops**, it's like your legs are glued together. Think of drawing a teardrop with your toes. Bend at your knees, and bring your toes down to the side on a diagonal. Circle at the bottom to bring your toes to the other side and up on an inward diagonal on that side to make the point of the teardrop. If you keep your hips fluid with this, they can move with the motion and add to the effect. Down, around, and up, drawing a teardrop with your toes.

The single-leg version of this move is very similar, but keep one leg pointed to the ceiling. The other leg crosses that leg on a diagonal, does its semicircle at the base, and comes back up to create the point. Then swap legs. The other leg crosses the straight leg, circles around, and comes back up.

I find that my knees and body don't flow as well with this option, so I do a half teardrop, which I also feel adds more energy. I go down on the diagonal, do my semicircle, then semicircle back, going back up the way I came. Options, options, options!

Let's look at the **single-leg teardrop**.

Step 1: Keep your toes pointed to the sky, legs straight.
Step 2: Bring one leg down on a diagonal across the straight leg.
Step 3: Semicircle across the bottom as if drawing a teardrop.
Step 4: For the full version, bring your leg back up diagonally. For the half version, don't go back up. Reverse the move, and semicircle back again.
Step 5: Swap legs.

Remember that fluidity in the hips makes this move much more flowy and gives more energy.

Straddles on the floor

Straddles can look really dramatic, but you'll feel it if you whack your ankle bones together! Instead, beat your feet at the top, crossing one in front, then behind. This creates a smooth flow, keeps energy, and provides an easy transition without the abrupt, dramatic, and painful CRASH of the ankle bones. Let's take a look.

Step 1: On your back, point your toes to the sky, keeping your legs straight.

Step 2: Bring your legs out to the side into a **straddle**.

Step 3: Bring your legs back together, crossing them over, one foot in front of the other. Try it one way, then the other (back and forth).

Now you can really jazz it up and go with the flow. Take a look at **straddles with flair**!

Tip: think of circling your toes in the direction you want your legs to go. Circle out to go out, and circle in to go – you guessed it – in!

Step 1: On your back, point your toes to the sky, keeping your legs straight.

Step 2: Keeping your knees together, bend at the knees to circle your toes in a full circle outward, then out to the side into a **straddle** (legs now straight).

Step 3: Bring your legs back together by circling your toes in a full circle inward, then together.

What I love about incorporating burlesque floorwork into pole routines is that you don't need to be in that exotic mindset. For me, lights, music, and atmosphere all help to create the exotic mindset, and if you aren't in that space, you feel like a right git! (Or at least I do!) Burlesque is satirical. It can be exotic, or it can be any character you choose. It can be fun and take the mickey out of things. It can be cheeky and playful. It gives a whole range, so you don't need to be in red-light-district mode. Once you have

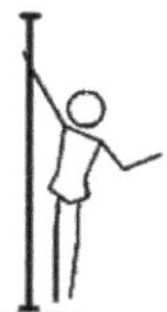

some foundation floor moves down, getting sensual is your choice. The trick of it is all about finding your 'safe-zone.' Find that mode, where you can be you, you can feel the music, you can feel the way your body wants to move. Switch your head off and flow. Whatever style that is, is unique to you, whatever is needed to create your safe zone is unique to you. If you need heels to flow, then great; heels open up so many doors for floorwork, like I said, you can slide on the toe of your shoe, or even clack it onto the ground, and not risk your toes (as long as your shoes fit right!). If that isn't you, that is fine too. But it is important to have a range of floorwork moves in your repertoire for those days where the pole slip is too much, fatigue hits, or if you are doing a pole show, and still need to finish the show- but can't do it on the pole, you can always finish it on the floor. It is just a case of finding your flow and style. You can find it on the floor, and then bring it up onto the pole- or bring your flow from the pole, down to the ground; just make it you!

Getting up off the floor... nicely

An ever-so important practice, and we have already looked at so many! Just in case you forgot some...The **peek-a-boo,** as you know, is one move that really adds to that feeling. It's playful, cheeky, and fun. Let's take another quick look.

Step 1: On your elbows, lean back. Point your toes to the sky, keeping your legs straight.

Step 2: Keep your toes together as you slide your legs down, knees coming apart.

Step 3: Peek-a-boo through the gap in your knees.

Step 4: Bring your legs back up to straight again.

Bow and Arrow (in floorwork)

Adding a little bit more sensuality to it, you have your **bow and arrow**. A **bow and arrow** move uses one leg bent, one straight. In pole, there are so many versions! The trick with this one is that the lower you allow your leg to go, the more ab work you're doing. The higher your legs are, the less abdominal strength is needed, so play it to your level.

I like to think of wearing a beautiful pair of stockings that you're rolling up or down with your feet or feeling with your toes. Starting on your back, if you're staying flat on your back, remember to pull your belly button down to the ground to remove the gap between your back and the floor. I think this move can be a lot more sensually dramatic if you're resting on your elbows. Lower one leg down straight as you slide the other toe up the straight leg. Then slide that toe back down the leg as you lift it up again. Now rotate, sliding the other toe down as you lower.

Step 1: Get in position on your back or elbows. Point your toes to the sky, keeping your legs straight.

Step 2: Keep one leg straight as you lower it down slowly.

Step 3: With the other leg, point your toe and bend your knee as it runs up your leg (towards the knee) as you lower. Steps 2 and 3 happen simultaneously.

Step 4: As you lift your legs, slide your tracing leg back down to the toe.

Step 5: Swap legs.

The Naughty Bounce

Now you're going to get on your knees for the **naughty bounce**. This move can literally look like you're thrusting the pole, so you need to add some class and style to jazz it up.

Have the pole right in front of you as you kneel, sitting back on your ankles. With one hand holding the pole for stability, bring your hips up to the pole, raise yourself up to a kneeling position, and come back down to sit.

Meet the thrust! This thing can look seriously un-classy. Here's the trick: watch your other hand (the one that isn't holding on to the pole). It starts on your lap, but as you bring your hips to the pole, bring it straight, hand posed flat with its fingers pointing out behind you. Now turn your head to look at it. As you come back down, bring your hand back to your lap. Suddenly, you've taken the focus away from the thrust and have created a beautiful shape, all while maintaining the sensual allure of the thrust.

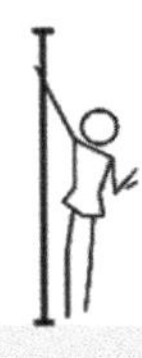

Personally, I prefer to body roll from this position instead of **naughty bouncing**. Sitting back on my knees, I bring my nose to the pole and rise up to bring my chest to the pole, followed by my belly. I then come back down to sit on my knees. I like the flow of this, but my body moves with a lot of curves, so it works well for me. These body rolls also allow you to smoothly transition to standing. Let me show you.

Step 1: On your knees, place your hands on the pole, sitting back on your feet.

Step 2: Bring your nose to the pole.

Step 3: Bring your chest to the pole as you rise up.

Step 4: Bring your stomach to the pole.

Step 5: Tuck your toes underneath you on the floor.

Step 6: Rock your hips back into a squat.

Step 7: Bring your nose back to the pole to body roll up to standing.

The Stripper Push-up

The **stripper push-up** can be made a lot harder than it really is, but it's a great way to get you down to the floor and back up again. The best way to think about it is body rolling onto the floor. Starting on your hands and knees, hands under your shoulders, knees under your hips, move your torso back slightly so that your hips come more over your feet (similar to a child's pose). Line yourself up, keeping your knees and hands still. You want to drift your body forward, leading with the head and bringing your nose down between your hands, almost touching the ground. Continue drifting forward as you move your chest through; forget hovering! Let your chest touch the ground, and slide forward until your belly is on the ground, straightening your arms and lifting your shoulders (similar to a cobra position).

To reverse this move, lower your chest back down. This is where you'll notice if you have one arm that's stronger than the other. You want to evenly push into the ground with both hands as you slide your bottom back again. I find it easier to have one knee bent with the foot pointing to the ceiling. This allows me to rotate over the knee, creating an easier pivot point and lever to work from. It's also a nicer shape.

This might sound a little confusing. Let's break it down.

Step 1: Down on the ground, on your hands and knees, push back so that your bottom is over your feet (like a child's pose).

Step 2: Bring your nose down diagonally between your hands, and move forward, one vertebra at a time.

Step 3: Bring your chest to the floor, and drag it along the floor.

Step 4: Bring your stomach to the floor as you drag forward. Push up with your hands to raise your chest up (cobra pose). Pose one foot to the sky, knee on the ground.

Step 5: Lower your arms to bring your stomach back down.

Step 6: Push evenly on your hands to slide your bottom back over your feet.

Step 7: Repeat!

This is a great move to use to roll onto your back. Once you've come through in the **stripper push-up**, as you lift your chest up, slide one arm out straight. You can now easily roll over that arm onto your back. Whichever arm you straighten will decide which way you roll. I recommend rolling away from the pole in most circumstances so that you don't get stuck with your subsequent leg work.

This has set you up for all your kicks and similar moves that we've covered so far. It has also set you up for a different way to get up: the **goddess rising**.

The Goddess Rising

For the **goddess rising**, start on your back, again with one leg bent and the other straight. The bent leg helps to create a smaller lever to come up to and looks much more posed and balanced. Think of the angle, lying down, torso to leg. It's like 180 degrees. Now bend one leg. The angle between your torso and that leg is a bit over 90 degrees. The smaller angle makes it easier to come up.

You want to think of having a string attached to your chest that is pulling you up, chest first. Your head comes up last. Perform this move without resting or putting pressure on your head or neck; this means relying on your abs!

To make it easier, put your hands flat on the ground and out to the side, in line with your shoulders. As that imaginary string pulls you up, use your hands, dragging them in with you but also pressing them into the ground. I find that if I apply slight

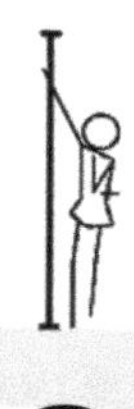

pressure along the pinkie side of my hand, it's easier to slide and apply pressure at the same time. (Be cautious as different floor coverings have different risks, carpet burn, splinters etc.) Once seated, look forward. This hand drag-in is totally dramatic, and it also makes the move much easier! Let's see it.

Step 1: On your back, bend one knee. Place your hands out to the side in line with your shoulders.

Step 2: Bring your chest up first as you press into the ground with your hands.

Step 3: Let your chest lead as you slide your hands in, pushing the sides of your hands to the ground.

Step 4: Once you're seated, look up/forward.

Okay, so it is a bit ridiculous, and it's a fair bit of work, but it looks and feels amazing when the flow is there! With your hands out to the side, gliding in, it gives a full luxurious satin-sheet-style feel – totally elegant!

If you're keen for an easier option, have your hands by your sides, fingertips pointing to your toes, just like if you'd been on your elbows doing **little kicks** and the **peek-a-boo**. Your hands should be flat on the floor at around waist height, with your forearms also resting on the floor. Let your chest come up first, as with **goddess rising**, but then rotate your weight onto your hands for the last part of the sit-up. Push up with your hands, then look up.

Here you are, sitting with one leg bent, one straight, beautifully posed, and it's easy enough to roll onto your bent leg for a crawl.

Crawls

Crawls are good to consider if you had too much fun with your floorwork and have ended up way too far away from the pole. If you stand up and walk back to the pole, it looks like you messed up. But if you **crawl** back, it's all part of the show! **Crawls** are very much a journey of personal discovery. Everyone's body moves so differently. Mine really rotates around the joints, so I take more of a lioness style. If your joints don't rotate as much, you can go long and smooth like a lizard. Whatever you do, don't prance around like a puppy or plop like a baby! It's all about light, deliberate moves, and I find that embodying an animal really helps with that. It feels and looks more "natural" by representing a creature that is already in existence, even if you do it in your own way!

With **lioness crawls**, I roll around my shoulder joints, letting my chest drop as I roll up and back around the shoulder joint, really exaggerating the movements, making them slow and primal.

Lizards are longer and flatter, reaching out long and sliding along with the opposite knee coming in as the arm reaches out.

Play with your style and how your body moves, and work out what works for you.

Levels are key!

Remember, playing with Dynamic levels in your routines not only maintains the interest of the audience but also mixes it up for you. As amazing as your spins may be, a whole song of spins can get lost. However, adding in some dynamic levels, different height moves, spins, floorwork, dance moves, it really mixes up the routine. Making it visually, more interesting. It also allows for each muscle group to rest and not get over-worked.

Also being able to put two moves together, and create routines is a completely different level of fitness. There is once fitness level for training moves, the next for routines. So having a mix of moves allows you to gradually build up your repertoire and combinations, one move at a time. Put two moves together- is that your limit? Okay, how to we take it to the floor? That is then a third move right there! Eventually you can have a more intense training session with a mix of moves to train and combinations.

When I taught rock climbing a fellow instructor told me to always try a different way of saying the instructions every time you run a lesson. That way, if you ever got a tricky group or client, you had a range of ways to try and make it work for them. The same thing applies here. Have a range of ways to combine moves, to get into floorwork, to get down to the floor. Mix it up, keep it interesting, and keep it safe. If you are ever feeling like you're stuck, you have options under your belt to try!!

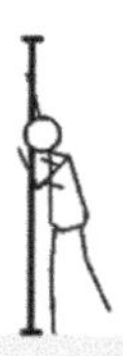

Discovering the History of Pole

Pole fitness started in a number of countries as a male-dominated strength-based sport. It turned to sensuality, then back to sport, evolving for all genders. There are so many stereotypes regarding pole, and this leads to many misconceptions. Understanding the roots of this sport is an integral part of acceptance of it. It has a history, and each step in that history made pole dancing what it is today.

Pole Sports: Tracing the Historical Influences by Ashley Wiggins[9] is a fantastic book if you're looking into the history of pole. Ashley has done very thorough study into the history of pole, looking not only from a pole sport perspective but also examining its growth through acrobatics, gymnastics, and yoga. She has traced the sport's origins back to the Silk Road, where the 7 major strands of pole sports originated. These include Chinese and Indian strands, as stated below, but pole sports later emerged in Japan as well.

To add some perspective to that, the Silk Road is a trade route that extends approximately 6,437 km (4,000 miles) through deserts and mountains. It's not one road; it's a network of routes used by traders since 130 BCE. Hundreds of festivals, displays, and ceremonies still take place every year along the Silk Road.

Pole fitness dates way back, with exotic pole, pole arts, pole theatre, pole sports, Mallakhamba, Chinese pole, and pole fitness all linking back to the Silk Road. Let's have a brief look at some of these origins and where styles have developed.

Africa

One of the oldest cultures in the world has deep-rooted traditions focused on sensual dance. Dance is an important part of African culture and is used for many rituals. It's not only a celebration performed at festivals and events like weddings; it also helps strengthen tribes in times of change or stress, and it brings people closer in times of joy.

Some African pole dances use props such as sticks to symbolise spears as well as smaller dancing sticks, depending on the reason for the dance. Such as a Zulu dance tradition for virgins to bring reeds to the king. The strength of the reeds is very important for this dance, as they symbolise virginity.

The Zulus also have an awesome wedding dance. The bride's family gives her away, and the groom's family accepts her. I have heard of a pole-related wedding ritual in some tribes, but I am yet to find evidence of this.

India

The Indians have a traditional high-energy acrobatic dance, which uses a wide wooden pole (these days around 55 cm at the base and 35 cm at the top) with a wooden edge. This apparatus has been said to have been designed for wrestlers to train on. In typical wrestler style, they use minimal clothing and no shoes, as this allows more skin to grip the pole, which is covered with castor oil to reduce friction.

Athletes achieve all sorts of amazing feats on the pole, as well as on top of the pole. These include flips on, off, up, and down the pole. Poles are used to develop speed, reflexes, concentration, and coordination. If that isn't enough, they also help with stamina, strength, and endurance.

There have also been studies done that prove training the rope variant of Mallakhamb is effective in developing optimism in children.[15] Mallakhamb is a traditional dance intended for male athletes and potentially dates back to the 12th century before being revived in the 19th century. Mallakhamb's name reflects its practice; 'malla' means 'wrestler' or 'gymnast', and 'khamba' means 'pole'. There are many versions of Mallakhamb, including plain, hanging, rope, and revolving bottle. Yes, you heard me right![12]

China

Dating back 1,000 years, Chinese pole has its own strength and balanced version, its techniques arising from tree-climbing in agriculture. This is where a lot of the extreme pole dance moves (like the **flag**) have been derived from in our modern style. Again, this is predominantly a male athlete sport, with lots of seamless climbing in many styles.

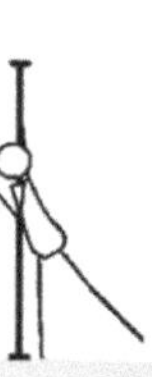

Generally, the Chinese pole artists use 3–9 metre rubber-coated poles, and pole dances are performed fully clothed. I'm not sure when sticky poles came in, but if you're not using a rubber-coated Chinese pole, there are also ones coated in a form of rosin to improve grip. If you've seen pole acts at circus shows, circus poles are generally Chinese poles.

Due to the clothing worn, Chinese pole is generally less fluid, but dancers have the ability to do quick drops down the pole and flips from one pole to another. This art form may be where the pride for pole bruises/kisses comes from, as in the past, performers regularly had pole burns on their shoulders or sides, depending on the drops and moves they'd done. This became a way for them to identify others and have respect for one another within the Chinese pole community.

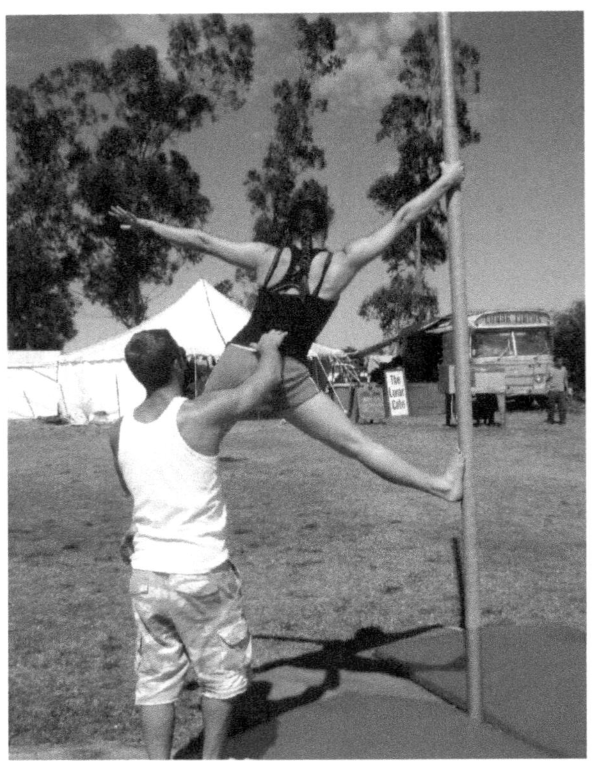

From my experience with Chinese pole, these are normally thicker poles – around 50 mm. Considering that you also wear shoes to help you climb, I suspect the extra girth of the pole helps with grip and the ability to clamp on to stop yourself in a drop.[17] If you think about pole dance, the thicker the pole, the more there is to grip onto, so leg grip moves become easier as there is more contact.

Medieval Europe

Pagan and Roman rituals of the maypole date back to the 12th century. Traditionally, with the Pagan fertility dance (given the phallic nature of a pole), girls would dance around a wooden pole, originally a living tree, with flowers and ribbons in a celebration of life. This is something you can see recreated at Renaissance fairs. It's less about dancing with the pole, more about dancing around the maypole. Some say that the hope of performing this act was to bring good fortune in marriage and to attract the opposite sex.

Many people say maypole dancing started in Germany. However, historian Helen Carr looked deeper into May Day celebrations, for which the maypole is iconic, finding that its origins seemed to be either Celtic or Roman and went far beyond dancing around a pole. The celebration was originally full of flames, burning the old to invite the new. Unfortunately, Carr found that the tree that was danced around for the maypole dance was then cut down and brought to town. Once in town however, it was decorated and treated with respect to continue the celebration of life.

As much as many people cite the maypole as an origin of pole dance, there was no real dancing with the pole. There was a pole present, nonetheless, as a feature of this tradition, leaving it up to you to decide if you see this as a free-flowing dancing influence or a coincidence.

Hoochie Coochie

We have 2 different styles and origins of hoochie coochie here, as it is sort of an all-encompassing term for several provocative belly-dance-like dances originating in the mid-1800s. Think of the old-school snake charming dances or Parisian cancan dancers at saloons. It does get quite provocative if you think of olden-day French dancers, being multicultural and learning Indian dances to dance at American (Chicago) fairs!

There are the stories of a lesser-known dancer called Little Egypt, who took it one step further at P T Barnum's grandson's bachelor party in 1896 when she took her clothes off![10]

Then came the African-American culture and the blues. Here, a hoochie coochie refers to a drunken woman's genitals. 'I'm Your Hoochie Coochie Man' by Willie Dixon and Muddy Waters is the perfect reference to this.

Putting those aside, I welcome you to the roots of what a lot of people see as pole dance these days. During the Great Depression in the USA in the 1920s, dancers had to use what they had at hand to entertain and make a living, and this included the pole in the middle of a circus tent as they emulated a mix of the Parisian cancan and Indian belly dancing.

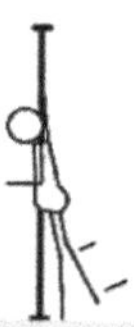

I can only imagine how important it would have been in such a dark time to have artists and entertainers brighten up the world a little! This style stuck and eventually grew in popularity. In the 1950s, it became a large part of the burlesque and cabaret scene as women expressed their sexuality.

Here, underwater striptease became a thing (riskily and unhygienically). Some stage shows got extra credit for not wanting to ruin their costumes in storms, performing in their bathing suits.[11]

Exotic Evolution

Exotic dance and striptease have a long history. From sacred rituals with Egyptian priestesses to the sun god Amun-Re to Mesopotamian cultures, many ancient cultures had sensual dances of seduction as offerings for their gods. Even mentioned in the Bible is the Dance of the Seven Veils, which has links back to the myths of ancient Sumerian times. The ancient Mesopotamian goddess of love, Inanna, danced, and as she did, she removed an item of clothing or a piece of jewellery at each of the 7 gates she passed on the way to find her love.

We also have the more well-known Moulin Rouge, which was notorious for its saucy dance numbers, as well as the ancient Middle-Eastern belly dance and the rumba and tango, all very sensual arts of dance.

In 1968, the first logged pole dancing case as we know it was performed by Belle Jangles in what was known as the Mugwump Strip Joint in Oregon, USA. This was the start of a new sport, though no one knew it. From there, the form grew, and in 1980, striptease and lap dance techniques started to be incorporated into pole dancing.

With an increase in risqué techniques came an increase in the popularity of pole dancing in Canada and the USA, bringing us through to the next milestone of the industry in the early 1990s.

In 1994, a lady called Fawnia Mondey/Dietrich was given a job as a dancer in Exotic Dance in Canada. Six months earlier, at 18 years old, she had sneakily glimpsed inside, seen girls dancing to 'In the Navy', and been inspired, but she got a shock. She hadn't realised how much weight she would lose when she took the job. This realisation linked with her passion for bodybuilding became her driving inspiration and led to her shift her focus at work to combining sensuality with sports moves, making pole dancing what it is today – something that people are fighting to have recognised as an Olympic sport.

Fawina established her own exotic dance school, and this also led her to create the first instructional DVD on learning the art of pole dancing. Multiple studios were opened across the USA by Sheila Kelley, who had been trained for a movie release in 2000.

There is a lot of focus on the USA and Canada in the birth of pole dance as we know it. Yet, strangely, as pole dance has evolved, it has been more readily accepted for its fitness benefits across the UK, Europe, and Australia than in the US and Canada, where there are still many stereotypes about what it is to be a pole dancer.

Today's Pole

Pole dancing today is a fusion of sensual western and eastern dance styles mixed with the energy and acrobatics of Indian pole and the strength and skill of Chinese pole. Thank you, Fawina, and the many others who followed, inspired, and developed this ever-changing industry!

When I started my pole journey in 2006, there were 2 studios in my state. The fitness studio I began at had beginner, intermediate, and advanced classes. Since then, I have lost track of how many times I have gone back to do the next level as it has come up. It has grown so much, and we have all grown with it, inspired by constant goals, each move being a new achievement, and achieving what we never thought possible.

We're still breaking down stereotypes and barriers, but we're doing it as a community that supports each other and grows together.

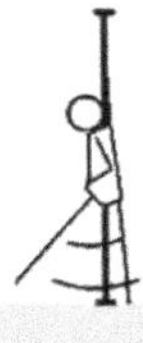

Bringing in the Obliques

By now, your shoulders should be quite stable. You've grown to know your grip, have stabilised your spins, and have even started to see how to move up slightly. Now you want to learn how to engage your obliques, your sides, and start playing with different angles. Once you're up the pole, these are amazingly important muscles, so you should have an understanding of how they work and move. Your best bet is to start early so that once you're up higher, stuff is starting to make sense.

The Basic Cradle

The **basic cradle** is a gateway move. It opens up many options for later on, so getting accustomed to using the muscles for the **cradle** is very helpful, provided you get used to it on the ground first. Once you have substantial strength in climbing and up-the-pole moves, this is one you can try up the pole too, along with its variations. It's much more oblique-y and a completely different motion to anything we've covered so far.

Basically, you're turning yourself into a sideways ball on the pole. Bring your outside hand across and onto the pole at shoulder height. Lean over so that your chest, staying side on, comes across to the other side of the pole. Now bring your bottom (inside) hand down in a **split grip** position with your index finger pointing down the pole. Create that push away triangle with your inside arm without sinking into your shoulder. (You will feel tension in your shoulder if your bottom hand is too high.)

If this hand is too close to the pole (or too low), pushing it will put pressure down the pole. You want to push the pressure onto the pole to create a solid triangle and a solid grip. This is usually about a 45-degree angle. From here, bring your inside leg up, bent at the knee, so that the thigh is pressing against the pole as close to the hip bone as possible. Get the pole up high; there is sort of a hip pocket spot here, and it's a handy thing to know. Ensure your shoulders are engaged, and solidify your grip before bringing the other knee up to join the first knee. Think of bringing your hips to the pole. Ensure your wrist is always aligned with the pole. Let's have a look.

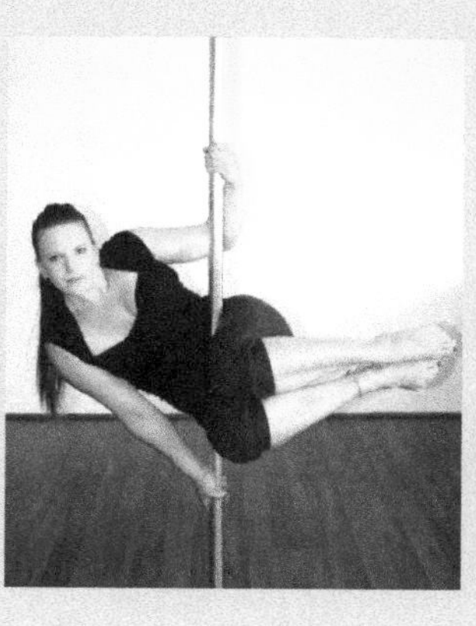

Step 1: Place your outside hand across, holding on at shoulder height.

Step 2: Bring your chest to the other side of the pole.

Step 3: Place your inside hand down to create your triangle grip, finger pointing down the pole.

Step 4: Bend your inside leg up, nice and close in your hip pocket.

Step 5: Stack your outside leg on top to join it.

Step 6: Reverse out of the move, controlling your legs first, you're your arms.

This move can be done spinning, and I must admit that it's a lot of fun. However, practise it static first until you get it right. That will help other variations of the move become easier without you needing to worry about leg placement. Once the move is solid and you're comfortable in it, feel free to try the spinning variation.

BASIC CRADLE GRIP

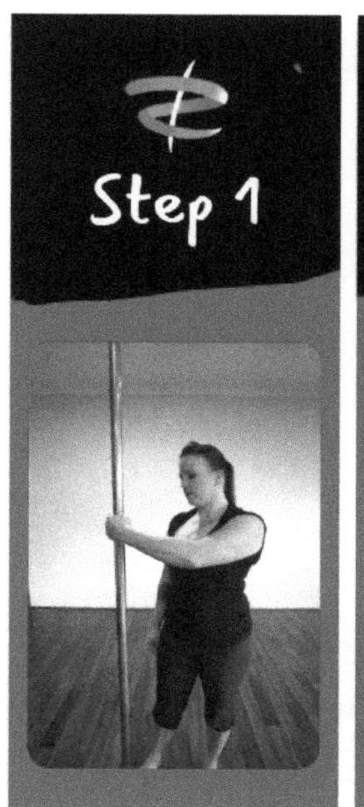

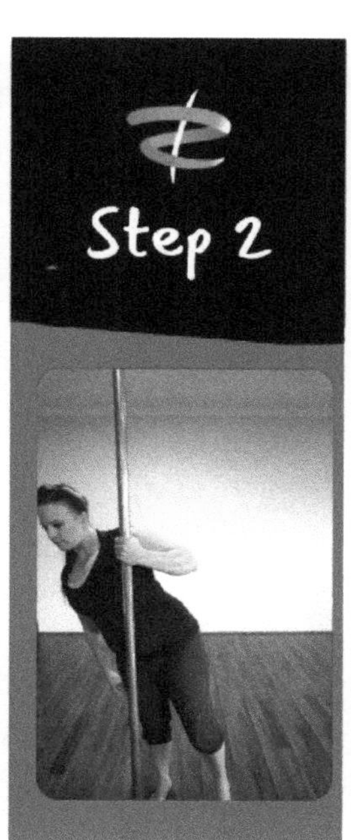

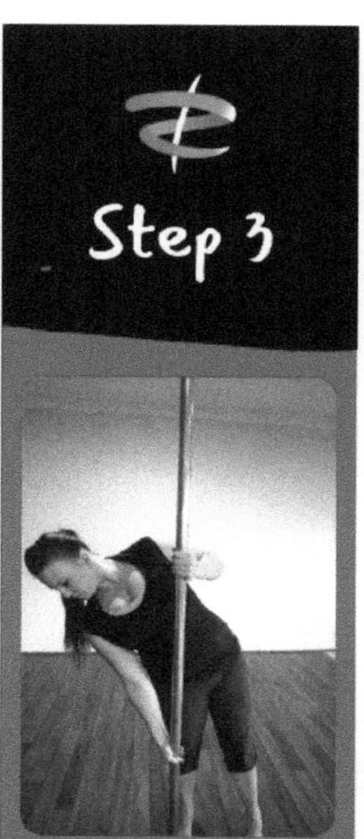

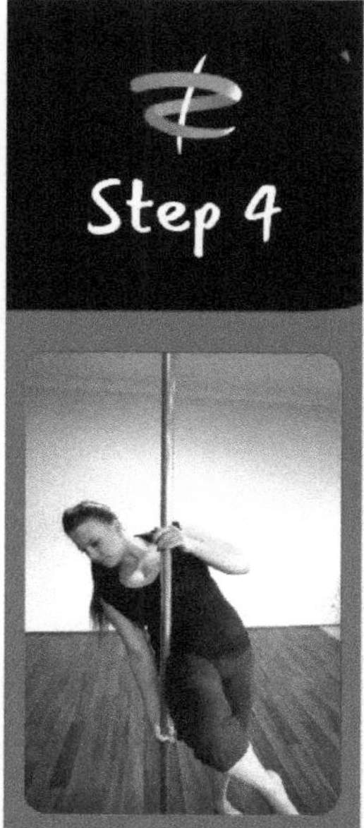

THE CRADLE

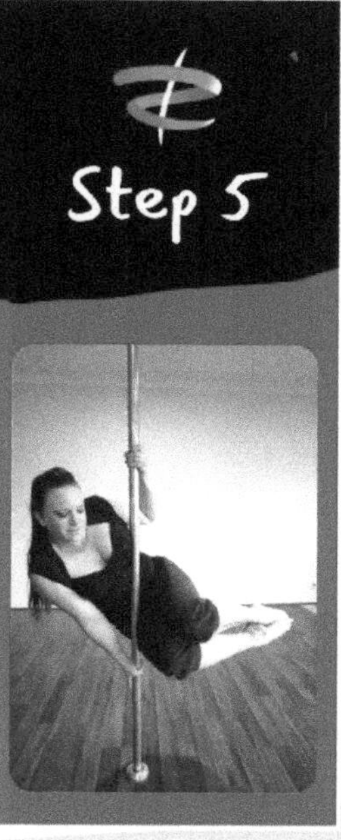

This is another foundation move that helps you advance and create flowing routines later on. It can transition you up the pole and can be a pose or a spin. Have a look at the QR code to guide you on your journey.

Muscles/Areas to Strengthen for the Basic Cradle

- Abdominals and trunk
- Biceps
- Shoulder girdle and scapular stabilisers (trapezius, serratus anterior)
- Rotator cuff (teres minor, infraspinatus)
- Latissimus dorsi
- Elbow stability muscles (if hyper-extensive in the elbows)

Muscles to Stretch for the Basic Cradle

- Pectorals
- Glutes
- Side (obliques)

It's time to have a look at some side-on spins. These use **split grip** to get you started. This can eventually prepare you for one-handed side-on spins. Adding in this sideways strength also helps you have more muscle control later when things get more inventive up the pole.

But for now, it's a whole new motion. Let's give a few variants a try.

The Peter Pan Spin

Start with the **Peter Pan**. Many of my students practise this thinking of a trotting horse, as it's a lot different getting your knees up high when not facing the pole. It's also a lot different not having the pivot into **split grip**. Let's give it a go!

Place your inside hand up high on the pole, shoulders rolled back to stabilise and help you avoid hanging from your shoulder joint. Stretch your outside hand across your body down low in a **split grip** position. Bring your outside leg up, knee in line with your hip, and push off with your inside leg.

I find that pushing through the ball of my foot keeps my (inside) leg straight. This leg then trails behind you. Keep facing forward as much as possible, trying not to rotate to the pole too much, although you do slightly. As per usual, doing the move with a walk is a lot easier than just lifting into it and attempting to create momentum. A good way to think about this is– crotch to the pole, not flashing the world!

Your outside knee is the one that goes up for this reason. If your back leg won't straighten, you can purposely bend it to stagger the legs (both legs bent at 90-degree angles, one in front of you, one below- also called "stag legs"), but if it's somewhere between straight and staggered, it looks like you're not getting the move. Going from a walk, let's give it a shot.

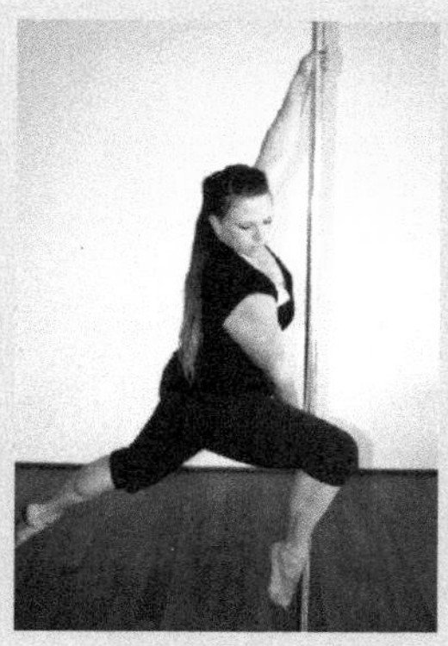

Step 1: Place your inside hand up, shoulder rolled back.

Step 2: Stretch your outside hand across in a **split grip** position. Pull with your top hand; push with the bottom.

Step 3: Bring your outside knee up nice and high.

Step 4: Push off your inside leg to straighten and spin.

Muscles/Areas to Strengthen for the Peter Pan

- Quads
- Hip flexors
- Abdominals
- Trunk extensors (erector spinae)
- Gluteus maximus
- Shoulder girdle and scapular stabilisers (trapezius, serratus anterior)
- Rotator cuff (teres minor, infraspinatus)
- Forearm flexors
- Elbow stability muscles (if hyper-extensive in the elbows)

Muscles to Stretch for the Peter Pan

- Glutes
- Hip flexors (with focus on rectus femoris)

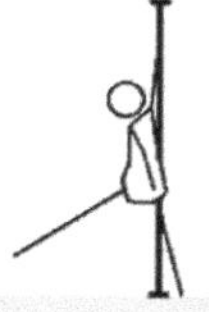

I hope you're still in the habit of practising everything on both sides! It's a good habit to get into after you have a move, practising your bad side first. As you spend more time on the first side you train, it gets your bad side better quicker. We have a QR code for this one too, a video to help you on your journey.

VISUALISATION: PETER PAN

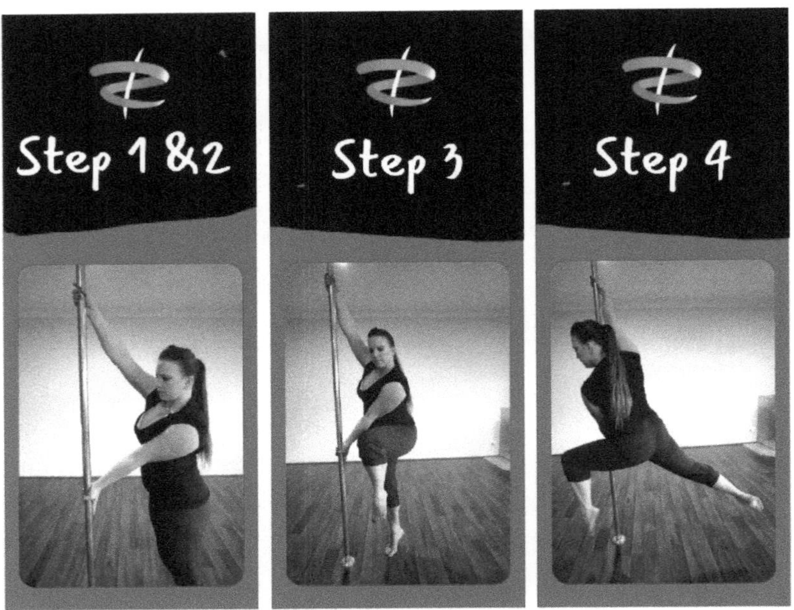

The Chair Spin

From a similar position, let's change it up for the **chair spin**. This one is a cute spin and is very similar. However, this time you start with your inside leg up first instead of your outside leg. This is because having your outside leg on the floor keeps your hips level and stable. If you bring your outside leg up first, it gives your hip a chance to dip and gives you a little stabilisation wobble as you start to spin.

After some practice, if you have the ab strength to stabilise your hips, you can start on either leg. I find it more natural to start with my outside leg, as most moves do, so with practice, after starting on the inside leg to get the move working for you, you can mix it up and find out whether you prefer inside or outside.

In the spin, you'll have both knees together and up as if you're going to sit on a seat. It does also require a fair bit of "push strength" with your outside arm.

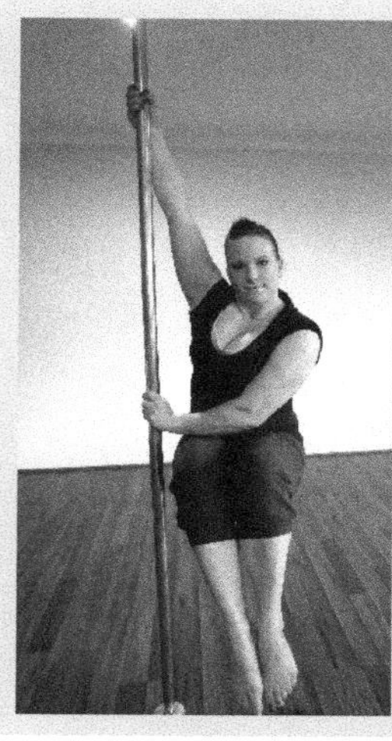

Step 1: Place your inside hand up, shoulder rolled back.

Step 2: Stretch your outside hand across your waist to **basic grip** (remember to push the pole away).

Step 3: Bring your inside knee up nice and high.

Step 4: Push off your outside leg to spin, and bring your outside knee up to join the other knee.

Step 5: As your spin slows, step and walk out of it.

Voila! You have it! Once you get comfortable in the spin, you can play with some variations. I have one variation that I really like. It adds a playful manner to the spin. From the **chair spin**, paddle your feet slowly, like you're dangling them in water. Keeping your knees together, slowly move your feet back and forth (as one goes forward, the other goes back). Just be aware of panic kicking; there's no need to turbo-speed kick! Keep a nice, calm, relaxed pace.

Muscles/Areas to Strengthen for the Chair Spin

- Obliques
- Abdominals
- Hip flexors
- Shoulder girdle and scapular stabilisers (trapezius, serratus anterior)
- Rotator cuff (teres minor, infraspinatus)
- Forearm flexors
- Elbow stability muscles (if hyper-extensive in the elbows)

Muscles to Stretch for the Chair Spin

- Glutes
- Hamstrings
- Lower back/lumbar

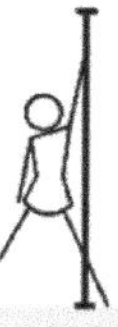

I find these side-on spins have a really nice feel to them and help solidify strength and grip for later one-handed side spins. But let's not get ahead of ourselves.

VISUALISATION: CHAIR SPIN

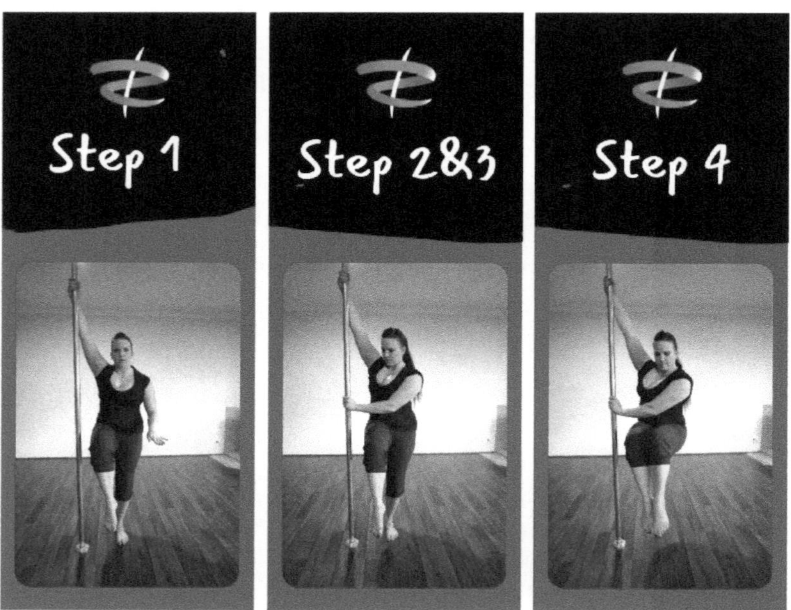

Low Pole Spin- The Low Lift Fireman

The **low-lift fireman** is one we've already started having a look at and doing the prep exercises for. Now it's time to turn it into a spin! As previously mentioned, I find **split grip** easier, as I like to have the space to see where I'm placing my feet, and it gives me more space to manoeuvre my legs without feeling too squished into the pole.

Please be wary of your elbows. Check if they hyperextend now that you've condensed yourself down at ground level. You'll need a bit of extra hip flexibility and a bit more ab and leg work to get your legs up and flat enough to make spins down here work.

Let's take a look.

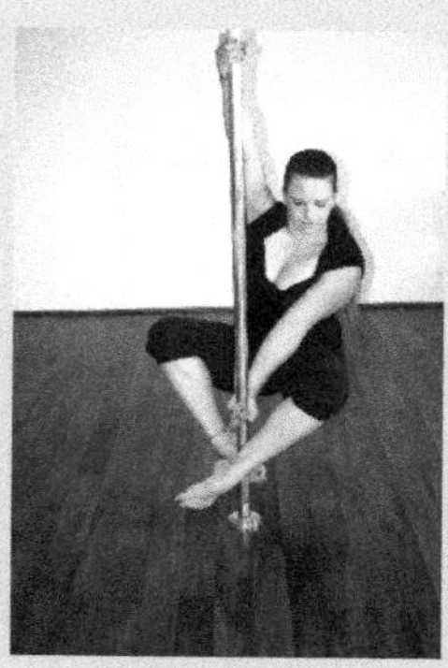

Step 1: Squat down, facing the pole.

Step 2: Straighten your outside leg out to your side.

Step 3: Place your inside hand up, palm facing the direction you're going. Roll your shoulder back.

Step 4: Place your outside hand down into your **split grip** as you slide your outside leg in a circle to the other side of the pole.

Step 5: Bring your outside leg in front of the pole (ankle to the front of the pole).

Step 6: Tap your other ankle to the back of the pole. Spin.

Step 7: Land on the balls of your feet, and continue momentum to stand.

Remember to practise both sides. You'll notice more of a difference down low. As there's less space for your limbs to flail around in, moves need to be more precise.

This move is a good introduction to low-pole moves. It's like a whole new world of pole dance! I generally relate it to climbing. Some people can climb up, while others find it easy to go sideways, also called bouldering. I go up! This means that low-pole flow confuses my body and doesn't work as well for me. If this flows really well for you, look into low-pole options, and see what's out there to find your style.

VISUALISATION: LOW-LIFT FIREMAN

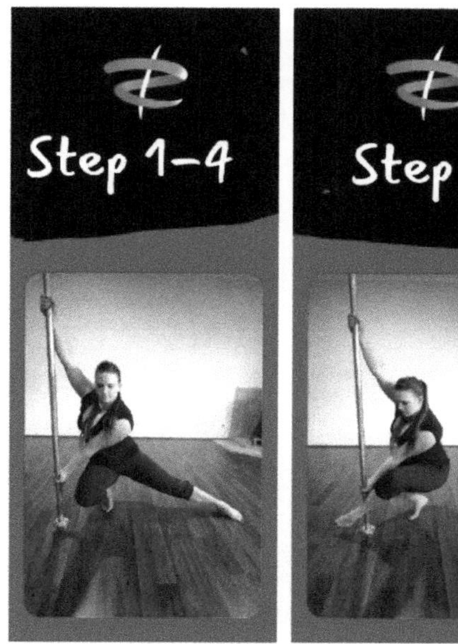

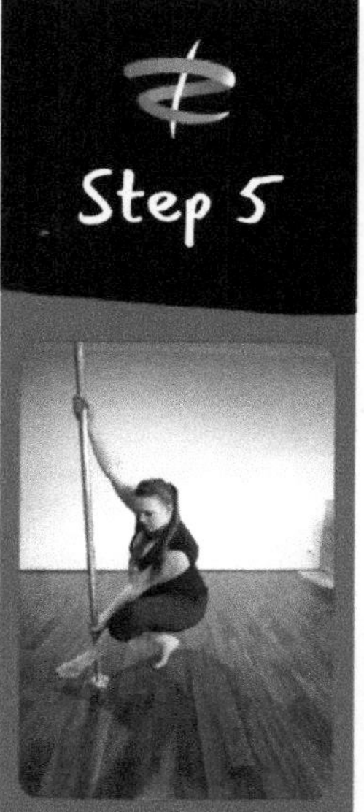

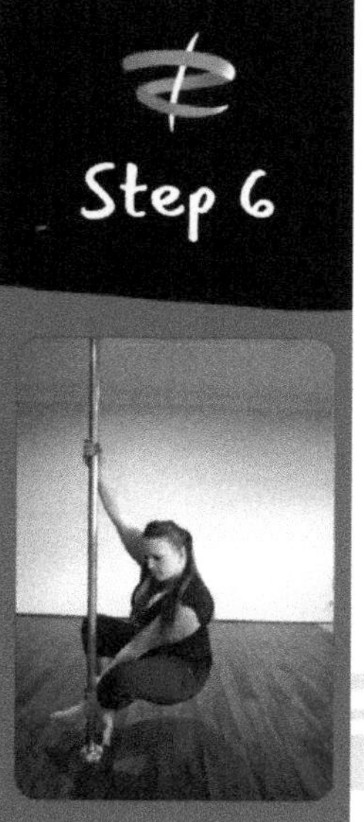

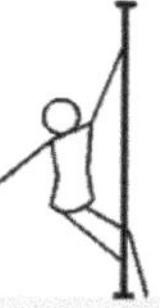

Girl Zone (sorry guys)

Training on Your Period

This is totally a personal preference thing. I've spent a lot of time talking about how everybody is different, and that's just as true here. The key is to listen to your body.

Symptoms range like no tomorrow when you're on your period, from bloating, cramps, and fatigue to feeling completely normal. Listen to your body. If you're feeling out of whack with lead feet, doing things with your feet above your head doesn't make sense. If you're feeling chirpy and bouncy, train whatever you'd like – safely.

Your period doesn't stop you from doing anything. Respect your body. It will tell you what it needs. But also embrace your femininity. It's a journey we all go through. Talking about it shouldn't be taboo; it should be natural.

I don't use tampons; my body just doesn't react well to them, so I swap between menstrual cups and pads, sometimes using both at the same time if I'm worried about a heavy day. Some days, I double up with underwear so no one sees the wings of my pad. Options are out there! Not everyone gets the chance to not work. Strippers, for example, tuck their strings in so that no one knows; they can't just take a week off every month!

Don't be afraid of your body. Be aware of it. Let it guide you. Be proud of your body, and if it's telling you to rest, let it rest. If it's a good week, continue on. There shouldn't be a problem pole dancing. The amazing thing about pole is how body aware you can become. It's such a gift, and it's empowering to feel like you know yourself inside and out!

We know the ins and outs of disposable pads and tampons. One of the issues with tampons is that they absorb the good stuff inside you so can cause irritations. This is something you are welcome to discuss with your health professional to find out what is best and what is happening in your personal situation. Both disposable pads and tampons, generally speaking, have all sorts of yucky chemicals in them, and some people will be more sensitive than others. If you find a brand that works for you, or that has less chemicals then that is an option for you to look at, there are also other potentially more sustainable options that you may or may not have considered.

There is the option of reusable fabric pads. If you're fine with blood, they are a viable option and are much more comfortable on the skin. Initially, with these, I wore double underwear until the pad moulded to my body and didn't move around anymore. I do still occasionally do this when training, depending on my attire. They do save you a lot of money, and you can still use these as a backup with things like the menstrual cup. Just remember to have some kind of bag for when you're out in case your pad needs changing. Keep something to put/wrap it in so you can pop it in your handbag without causing a mess like something out of a horror film!

As for menstrual cups, get the hang of the messiness of inserting/removing in the toilet or the shower, and learn to look after and sterilise them. They do help with period odour paranoia. If you're younger, having not had sex before can make these a bit trickier. There are latex-free ones, so if you have issues with latex, keep an eye out for silicone cups. Mensural cups are awesome for training, as there is no pad "wings" or strings to worry about.

Another option is period pants. I'm keen to try these out! I have friends who say they can lounge around without any spillage. You still have normal period odour with these, and if it's a heavy day, be aware that you may need to change your underwear throughout the day.

Kristy Sellars does some amazing work, telling stories with her pole choreography and really putting together the whole package when it comes to performances. Being immersed in the industry and having a passion for the environment, she also creates eco-friendly pole products. One of which is Period Pole Pants. Cheeky cut, high waisted, stylish, yet designed with an extra-wide crotch, not only for absorbency but so that you can move on the pole comfortably without worries. I am sure there will be many more advancements from all over the industry, but it is great to hear of long-term polers trying to solve those problems that many of us have and looking at what peoples' needs and concerns are to create a pole-specific solution.

There are bound to be more options. Flow with your body; it almost has a 'natural intelligence' listen to your symptoms. Remember to do your research, if need be, ask a healthcare professional about the best option for you.

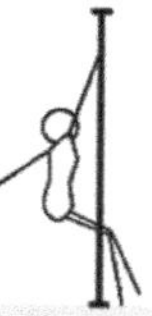

Returning to Pole Fitness after a Baby

Please heed your doctor's advice. There is a reason they say not to return to exercise until at least 6 weeks after birth, but the length of time before returning to exercise not only depends on the type of labour/birth that you had, it also depends on your fitness levels before pregnancy/birth and what you want to get back into.

Your body has been through an ordeal! Getting into things too soon can do more damage than good, and core, pelvic floor, and posture issues can hinder your return to pole for longer than necessary if you try to jump in too soon. Ask your physio or doctor, and explain your situation, your training regime, and your hopes for returning to training. Discuss timelines. If you're specific about your goals, your doctor will hopefully be more likely to offer recommendations.

Be realistic, though. Yes, starting from scratch can be frustrating, but if it's the difference between starting and not starting, the beginning is a good place to be! Don't forget to allow yourself time to recover. Let your body get back to its normal state before forcing it back to your desired normal when it just isn't ready yet.

Your Journey

**From my personal experience with 2 children. I am not qualified in this area.*

1. Pelvic floor! Get those muscles strong. I used to have a sticky note above the stove so that every time I was stuck mixing things or cooking dinner, I could do my pelvic floor exercises.
2. Your deep core will need strengthening and realigning.
3. Work on returning your abs to the right length.
4. Fix up your posture now that your weight ratios have shifted again.

Remember, your ligaments and soft tissue have all softened to allow for pregnancy and childbirth. You don't want to push them too far too soon! This is something to really consider. Everything became soft and floppy to allow the growth of a baby. Now that the little stowaway has arrived, that doesn't mean that everything goes SPRINGING back to normal. Those 6 weeks after birth are for rest and recovery. The last thing you want is a newborn and an injury!

Exercises to consider

1. Do whatever your physio says. Most hospitals allow you access to a physio after you have a baby. Follow their recommended exercises. Every pregnancy and labour experience is different, and every journey to recovery is different. Everyone's body is different.
2. Use wall angels to realign posture and assist with shoulder strength and function. Place your shoulders and bottom against the wall, feet a few inches forward, and keep your spine neutral. Place the backs of your hands on the wall at shoulder level, and slide them slowly up and down the wall as far as is comfortable, maintaining a neutral spine – no arching your back!
3. Try pelvic floor breathing to restore the connection between your core, diaphragm, and pelvic muscles, allowing you to create and release tension and regain muscle control. With a neutral spine, lie on your back with your knees bent, feet flat on the floor. Place your hands on your rib cage, and breathe in and out, feeling your ribs and stomach rise and fall. As you exhale, pull up through your pelvic floor, bringing your belly button to your spine. Imagine that you're pulling your hip bones together, and hold while breathing normally.
4. Do pelvic floor exercises. Find a way to remind yourself to do them. Leave a note on the bathroom mirror, reminding you to do them when you brush your teeth. What's going to work for you? Set a limit, a number to do, and make it achievable. Too much will put you off, so don't start on the back foot!
5. Do hip tilts to improve core function, range of motion, and stability in your posture with your pelvis and lower back. Sit tall on a fit ball with your feet hip-width apart and flat on the floor. You're going to make a very small movement. Tuck your hips under to roll the ball slightly towards your feet. Then, going the other way, roll the ball away from your feet. Repeat.

Changing It Up with Back and Abs

I like to focus on a similar range of moves each session, there is the need to re-cap what we have done before, but I like to know that I am warming up and stretching for a certain few moves in particular. Putting too many of the same types of moves together can lead to fatigue, but putting a couple in allows you to not only get accustomed to the motion, the grip, the muscle activation, it is like each one builds off the last, and it helps your brain and your body get acquainted almost with that style move. It also helps you know what to prepare for when you are warming up. Here is a different way of moving again. A lot more activation of muscles in your torso, but also a need to squeeze "the juice" (your bottom, or gluteus muscles). Now that we are more solid in our grip, we can play with a few different body positions. Let's begin…

The Carousel Spin

The **carousel** is a lot of fun. It's almost like a **straddle** but totally opposite. Basically, you're going to work on spins facing the pole directly, again involving completely different muscle activation. Your abs are extended more, your back muscles activate, and it feels totally alien.

Essentially, what you're going to do is start in your **split grip**, but instead of bringing your legs in front, they'll stay bent behind you. Getting into it isn't so complicated either.

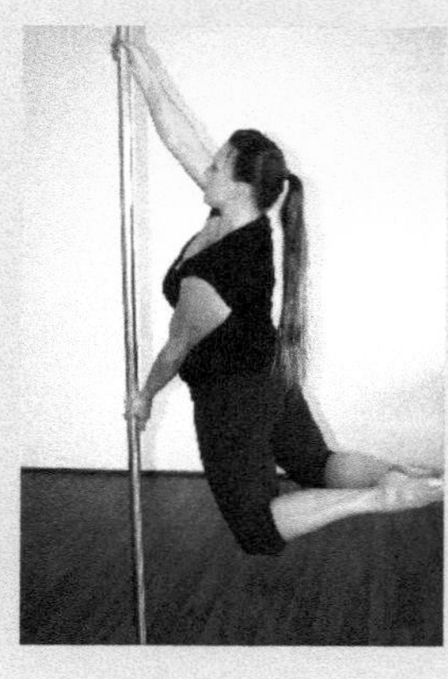

Step 1: Roll your shoulders back. Place your inside hand up, palm facing the direction you're going.

Step 2: Step on your inside leg. Pivot to face the pole.

Step 3: Place your outside hand on the pole with your finger pointing down the pole.

Step 4: Bring your outside leg up, bent at the knee as you pivot, leaving it there (right behind you at the pivot point). Pull with your top arm; push with your bottom arm.

Step 5: Push off your inside leg as you bend it (pointing toes together if you wish). Spin.

New muscles; new movements. I think that calls for another QR code, don't you? Have a play, and enjoy!

Muscles/Areas to Strengthen for the Carousel Spin

- Hip flexors
- Shoulder girdle and scapular stabilisers (trapezius, serratus anterior)
- Rotator cuff (teres minor, infraspinatus)
- Forearm flexors
- Elbow stability muscles (if hyper-extensive in the elbows)

Muscles to Stretch for the Carousel Spin

- Glutes
- Hamstrings
- Lower back/lumbar

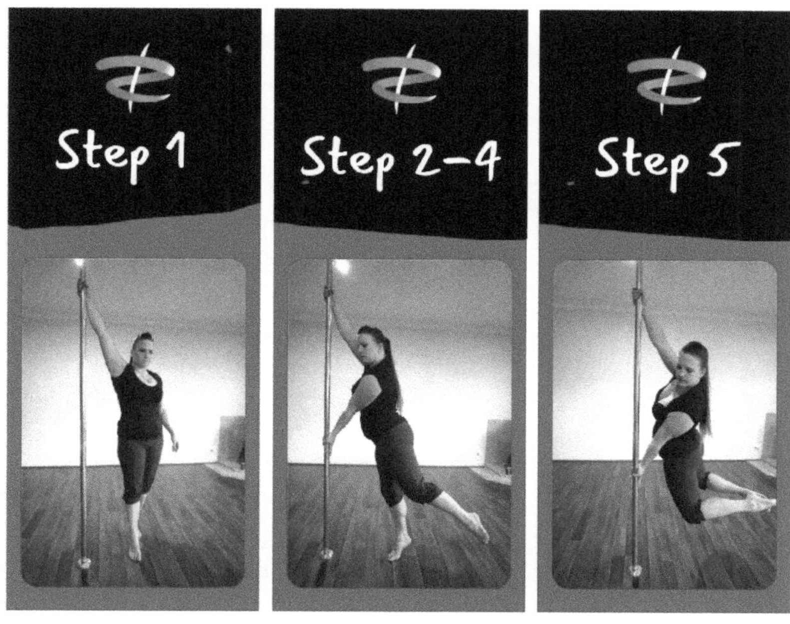

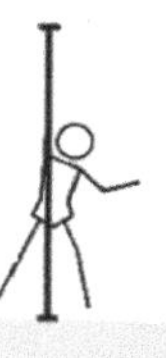

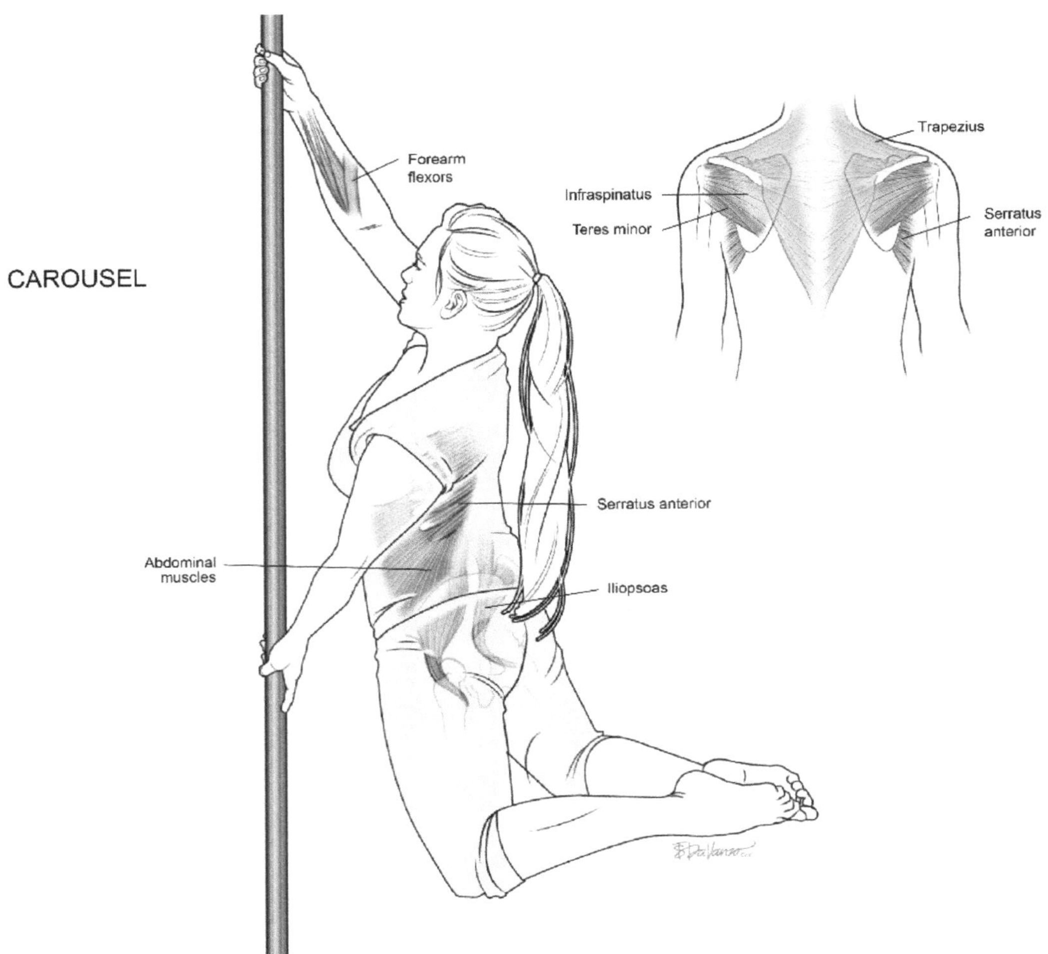

There is another more banana version of the **carousel**. This variation starts off exactly the same but is a little different in the muscles you squeeze to hold it. You really want to squeeze your bottom! Why Banana? Because this time our legs are almost... straight.

Step 1: Roll your shoulders back. Place your inside hand up, palm facing the direction you're going.

Step 2: Step on your inside leg. Pivot to face the pole.

Step 3: Place your outside hand on the pole with your finger pointing down the pole.

Step 4: Bring your outside leg up, allowing it to follow as you pivot, keeping it straight, leaving it there. Pull with your top arm; push with your bottom arm.

Step 5: Push off your inside leg as you bring your legs together and spin.

Muscles/Areas to Strengthen for the Straight-Leg Carousel Spin

- Hip flexors
- Shoulder girdle and scapular stabilisers (trapezius, serratus anterior)
- Rotator cuff (teres minor, infraspinatus)
- Forearm flexors
- Elbow stability muscles (if hyper-extensive in the elbows)
- Gluteus maximus
- Hip extensors

Muscles to Stretch for the Straight-Leg Carousel Spin

- Hamstrings
- Rectus femoris
- Lower back/lumbar

This banana-body variation is also in the previous QR code.

The Pole Slide

The **side-pole slide** is one you need to be careful with, especially if you have hyper-extensive elbows. You can do **basic grip** with this if you're concerned. However, I find you feel more stuck on the pole, and it gives you less space to move than in **split grip**. The trick is getting used to a safe release without putting too much pressure on your grip, especially your bottom arm.

In **split grip**, stagger your feet out to the side and, bit by bit, edge your feet out so that you can slowly release your grip evenly with your body. Slide down as far as you can before bending your back leg and sliding into jazz splits.

What? Splits? Jazz splits! Basically, if the front leg is straight and the back leg is bent, from the front, it gives the illusion of splits. Voila! Jazz splits!

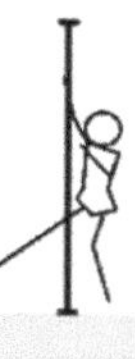

Please don't push your body more than you're able to. Slide down, using your feet to assist so as not to strain your upper body. Don't force the split, and ensure you have thoroughly stretched prior to this move.

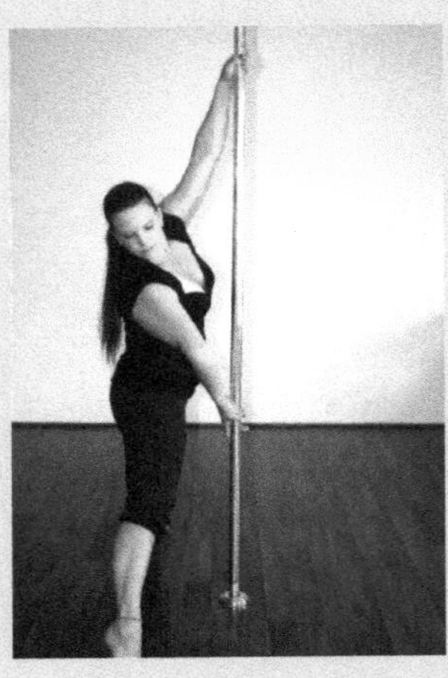

Step 1: Roll your shoulder back. Place your inside hand up.

Step 2: Place your outside hand on the pole with your finger pointing down the pole. Push and pull down the arms, pressure coming from your shoulders.

Step 3: Stagger your legs to the side, and start edging them out.

Step 4: When you're down as far as you can go, bend your back leg, and sit your bottom back.

Muscles/Areas to Strengthen for the Pole Slide

- Hip flexors
- Abdominals
- Quads
- Shoulder girdle and scapular stabilisers (trapezius, serratus anterior)
- Rotator cuff (teres minor, infraspinatus)
- Forearm flexors
- Elbow stability muscles (if hyper-extensive in the elbows)

Muscles to Stretch for the Pole Slide

- Hamstrings
- Adductors
- Hip flexors

VISUALISATION: POLE SLIDE

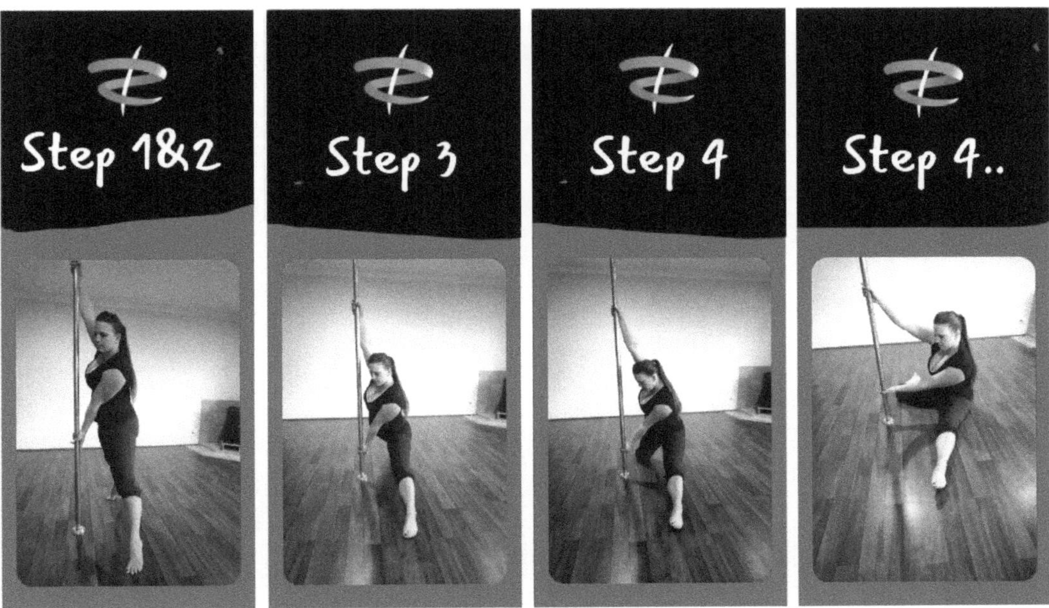

The Basic Teddy

Now it's time to have a bit of fun and look a bit more dramatic with the **basic teddy,** or **lifted straddle**. Here, you're trekking back to your **windmill grip** (the **basic invert grip**). This grip is going to stabilise you once again. Bring your hips in front of the pole, engage your abs and quads, and lift into a **straddle**. It's that easy!

This may take some time and practice. You can practise bringing one knee up first, then swapping to the other knee. Alternatively, you can try bringing both knees up into a tuck. But I find it fun to try the straddle. Don't stress about the height of your legs initially; that comes with time. You may surprise yourself that you can actually pull this off, especially if you've been practising the moves we've done so far.

Remember, the force of a jump going up, pulls you back down. Set your grip, stabilise, activate and lift! Activate your muscles and lift, not jump, into this move.

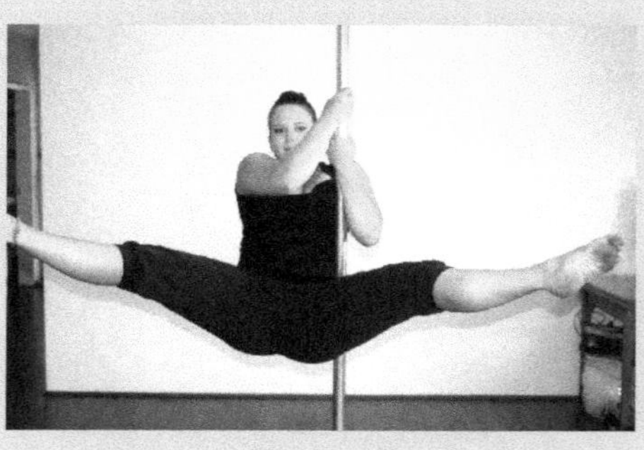

Step 1: Wrap your inside arm around the pole, holding on at face height, elbow down.

Step 2: Place your outside hand also at face height.

Step 3: Squeeze your inside arm onto the pole.

Step 4: Bring your hips in front of the pole, resting on the pole.

Step 5: Lift into a straddle.

Step 6: Step your legs down before your arms give in.

Then try the other side. Stand on the other side of the pole, and see how that goes. As hinted by the name of the grip, this is a good move, along with the **windmill**, to get you accustomed to the grip and slight lift to move up to your invert eventually. With practice of this move, you'll notice that you can lift your legs higher than before. Once you get control and feel comfortable in the move, you may even be able to slightly lean back and give the illusion of more flexibility as your hips tilt.

Muscles/Areas to Strengthen for the Basic Teddy (Lifted Straddle)

- Front line (trunk, abdominals)
- Scapular stabilisers (trapezius, serratus anterior)
- Hip flexors
- Quads

Muscles to Stretch for the Basic Teddy (Lifted Straddle)

- Hip adductors
- Hamstrings
- Lower back/lumbar

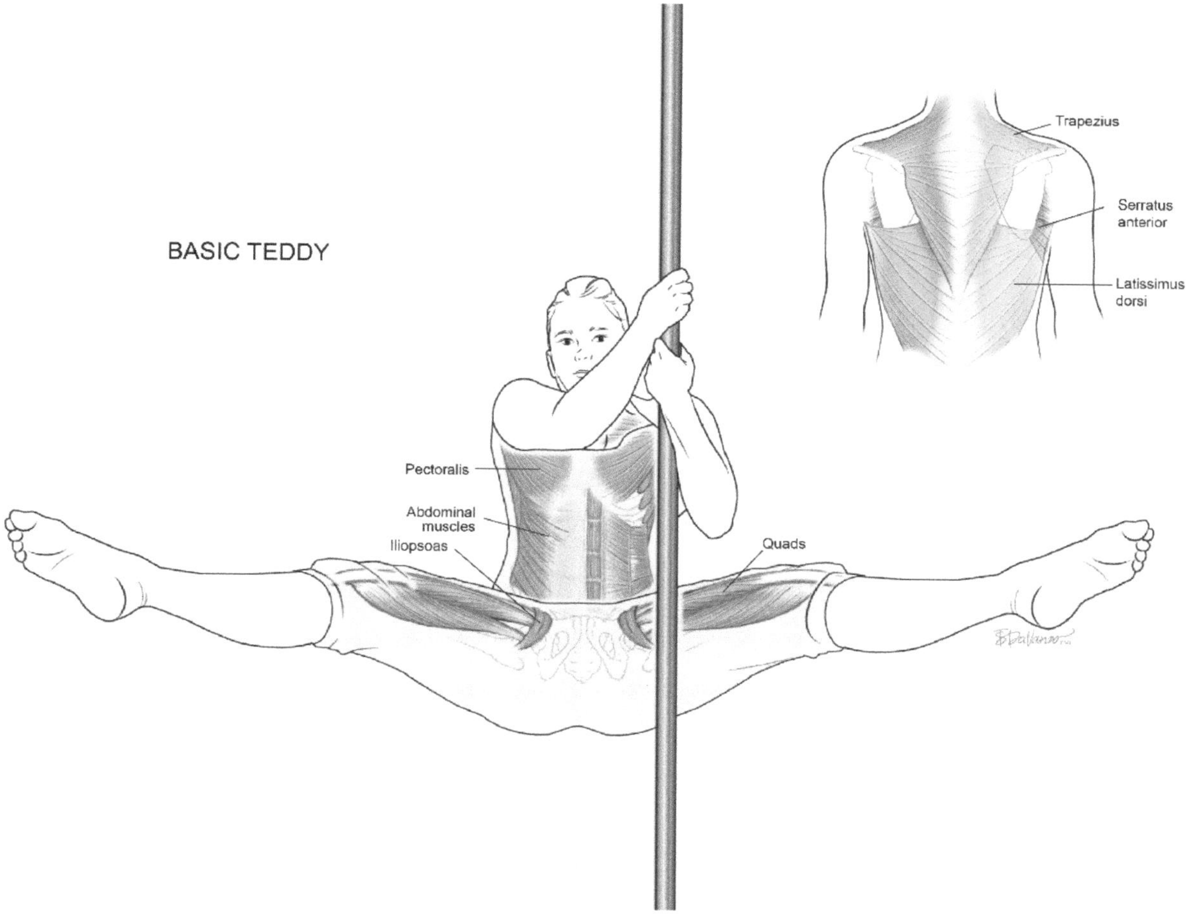
BASIC TEDDY
Trapezius
Serratus anterior
Latissimus dorsi
Pectoralis
Abdominal muscles
Iliopsoas
Quads

VISUALISATION: BASIC TEDDY

Step 1&2
Step 3
Step 3.5
Optional Tuck
Step 4..

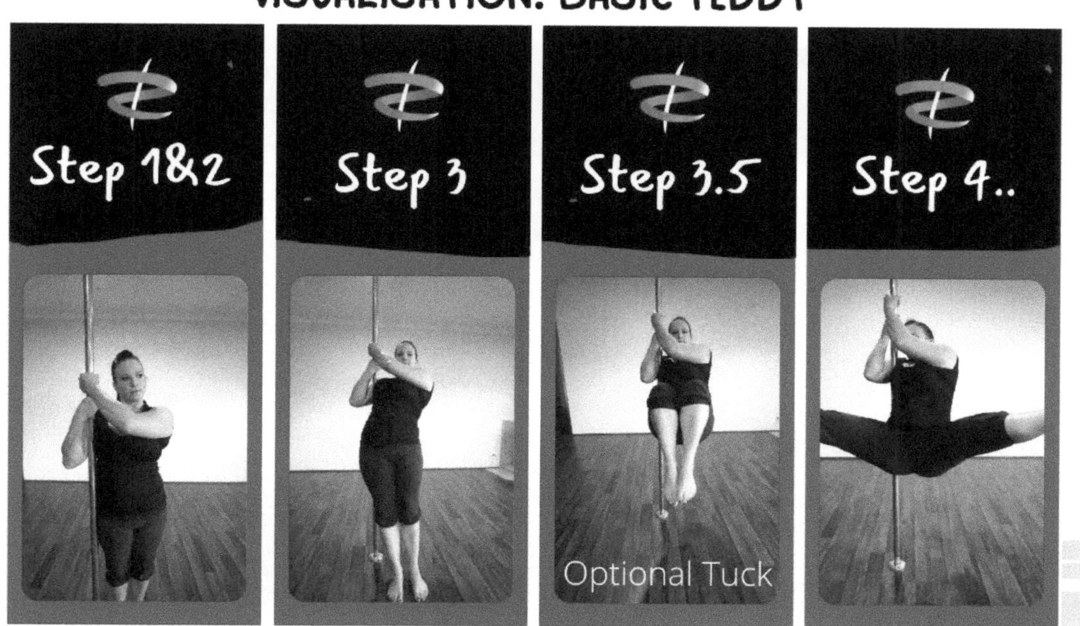

The Swan

The **swan** is an interesting move and is elegant on a spinning pole. Basically, it's a pose on a static pole. Try and spin it on a static, and the pole pinch is not pleasant! You can, however, use it as a slide down if you're on static. This is the reverse of the **backward spiral**.

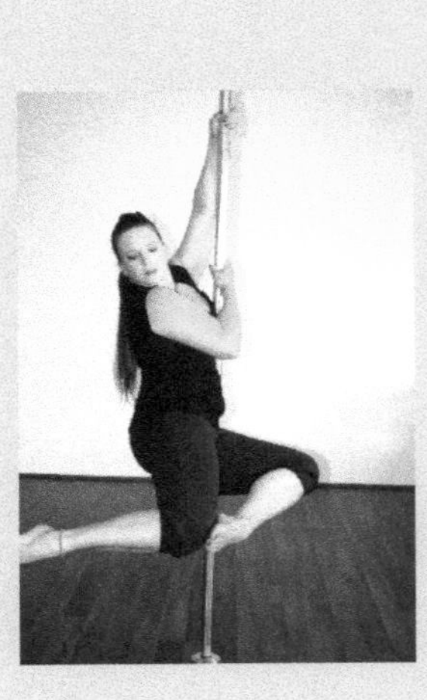

Step 1: Place your inside hand up, palm facing the direction you're going. Roll your shoulders back.

Step 2: Stretch your outside hand across your body, holding on at chest height.

Step 3: Bring your inside leg up onto the pole, resting it on your upper thigh (or hip pocket, where the quad/thigh and hip join).

Step 4: Bring your outside leg up behind you so that your front toe is pointing to your back knee. There's a fair bit of oblique/side lift here to get your legs flat.

Step 5: Hold! (Or spin on a spinny pole!)

Remember to train both sides and find your flow. Which moves work for you, and which moves don't? Pick your 2 favourite moves, and find a way to flow one into the other. Then pirouette and try the other side! Enjoy the journey and all the moves you now know!

Maybe even try to take a video, look at your lines, how you start, finish and transition into moves. Then try to make it smoother, creating good habits early by looking and posture, lines and positioning (even upon landing) will help you so much on your journey.

Muscles/Areas to Strengthen for the Swan

- Gluteus medius
- Abductors
- Trunk (abs, obliques)
- Shoulder girdle and scapular stabilisers (trapezius, serratus anterior)
- Rotator cuff (teres minor, infraspinatus)

Muscles to Stretch for the Swan

- Hip flexors
- Side (obliques)
- Hip adductors

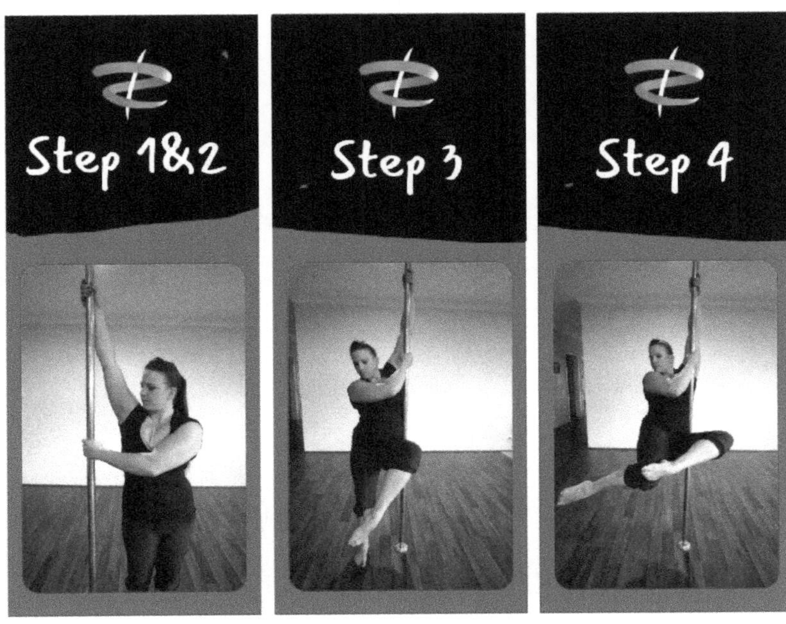

Learning the Science of Pole

That effortless look when you perform something tricky but make it look easy comes from a true understanding of your body and its movements. Really, it's all in the physics of it! If you have a basic knowledge of the physics of movement, you can jump higher, spin faster, move more quickly, and flow like liquid through your movements.

1. **Definition of physics**[19] (Merriam-Webster Dictionary Online. n.d)

   1: a science that deals with matter and energy and their interactions.

   2a: the physical processes and phenomena of a particular system.

   b: the physical properties and composition of something.

Let's put things in a physics perspective. Motion is one of the key topics in physics. Motion is a change in position of a thing with respect to time. Time passes; it moves. But even the slightest movements count. If you stand still, the earth is still rotating, so there's still motion. The movement never ends.

Add mass into that. Quite simply, anything of substance is made of matter and thus has mass. So far, for pole dancing, we have a mass in motion. Let's look at that a bit deeper.

Force

The harder you throw it, the harder it hits. The higher you jump, the faster you come down. Logical, right? Then why do our brains seem to be hardwired to jump into pole moves when we can use physics to help us?

The force we use to jump up is also going to pull us down, so let's not! There's that force word again. What is it? So we have a thing, anything. A force is any influence that affects or changes that thing – its shape, direction, or speed.

We can use velocity, momentum, and centre of gravity to assist. To do a spin, you need to use your body weight, or your mass, to create a steady motion in one direction around the pole. That's velocity. To do this, you move your centre of gravity, using different pushes, pulls, and swings (or forces) to help get your body off the ground, creating momentum.

Definition of force[19] (Merriam-Webster Dictionary Online. n.d)

1. strength or energy exerted or brought to bear; cause of motion or change; active power.

Thank you, Newton! His second law sort of sits in here. F=ma with lots of big technical words, meaning that the net force upon an object is equal to the rate at which the object's momentum changes. If you have a scientific brain, you're probably cussing me right now, but hopefully, it also helps a little. If not, an old, really influential dude said so!

Centrifugal and Centripetal Force

Centrifugal force is created by weight being flung around in a circle. Yay for pole! There are debates about this force being fictitious because, as much as you may feel the force pulling you, from someone else's perspective, it may look as if you're getting pushed. Either way, you feel your body being pulled from the centre. Add some momentum and velocity to that, and the pull increases, keeping you up longer. Make sense?[18]

Confused? Let's make it worse. I've included the technical force names, but forget them. Just think of the concept.

Centripetal force is a different type of force; centripetal force is a force which directs an object to move in a curved or circular path, this path has an inward focus. If you're tucked in close to the pole, you spin faster. The further away you are, the more you start to slow down. Centrifugal force is the apparent outward force that draws, in this case, a body away from the pole or the centre of rotation – that feeling of going so fast that it pulls you out. Start out from the pole, create the forward force/momentum/velocity, and it will help hold you out and up for longer.

Velocity

Basically, velocity is the speed that something moves in one direction. Think of spinning on a swing set. How can you speed yourself up or slow yourself down by bringing your body closer in or further away?

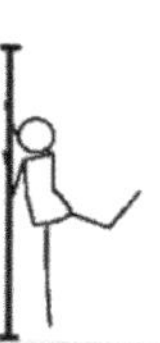

Definition of velocity[19] (Merriam-Webster Dictionary Online. n.d)

1a: quickness of motion: SPEED.

b: rapidity of movement.

c: speed imparted to something.

Centre of Gravity

We all know that what goes up must come down. But if you think a bit more about it, things that aren't just straight up and down can topple over unless they're perfectly balanced. Meet the centre of gravity (sometimes referred to as 'centre of mass').

That central point aligns everything to equal and evens weight distribution on either side. When you're hanging your body off the side of a pole, it's kind of good to have an understanding of this. It's not being aware of just your centre of gravity but also of the way this lines up. This helps you achieve smooth transitions, especially as you transfer your weight from one pole position to another. You need to be conscious of how gravity works.

Put simply, your centre of gravity is your point of balance, however this may align. All axes pass through this point; all the forces seem to act. Looking at the extreme, balancing on a tightrope, if your centre of gravity is anywhere BUT above the wire, you go splat! Your centre of gravity must be directly above that wire. Common sense, right? But there's so much more to it.

You know what's tricky? With an advanced move like the **ayesha** (think of a straddle spin, but as an upside-down hold, no spin), the centre of gravity may not even be on your body. You need to find that right level of push back with your hips, not only to align all your muscles and joints safely but also to find your centre of gravity to lock in and stay put.

Talking about alignment, there's also a line of gravity. This passes through the centre of gravity and is basically a straight line where force is distributed. You'll notice that your pole moves will partially travel in this line, or else they will feel unstable. You balance this line with your support spots (points of contact on the pole).

You may notice that having a support base in the lower body makes you feel like there is security and more movement available. Your upper body may feel like it requires more muscle control to maintain. The wider your base support, the easier it is to balance; the narrower your base support, the more muscle control is required.

Put your awareness of gravity to use. Do you need to be lower to have better balance in your flow moves or land a move with a wider stance? Pretty much every sport involves being aware of where your weight is and how to move it swiftly and smoothly without losing control or using too much energy. A basic understanding of your centre of gravity makes a world of difference.

Gravity has other fun pointers, like where you're attached to the pole. Is the mass of your body above or below that? Standing up on the pole looks very similar to the inversion crucifix (just to help picture the crucifix, imagine having your legs wrapped around the pole, upside down, with the pole running down the front of your body, and your arms out to the side). However, you feel less stable standing, as the bulk of your body is above your attachment point, whereas in the crucifix, the bulk of your body is lower, so there's less balance and more pull on your grip point by gravity.

Momentum

Any object moving will continue moving unless it is interfered with. Thank you, Sir Isaac Newton!

Basically, momentum is the speed (or velocity) of a moving object. The amount of momentum you get is dependent on the mass that's moving and how fast it's moving. Bringing a hand slowly to the pole doesn't give you much momentum, but swish a leg around, and the speed will affect the momentum you gain.

Angles also change which way you move. Make your momentum travel in that direction. Swishing your leg diagonally to go straight forward doesn't work, as your muscles put a halt on what you're doing to realign the movement.

Definition of momentum[19] (Merriam-Webster Dictionary Online. n.d)

1: a property of a moving body that the body has by virtue of its mass and motion and that is equal to the product of the body's mass and velocity.

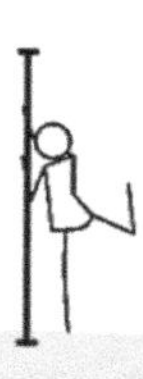

broadly: a property of a moving body that determines the length of time required to bring it to rest when under the action of a constant force or moment.

We use momentum with pole to start spinning and allow us more spin before friction finally slows us down. The more points of contact with the pole, the more friction and the quicker we slow down. Combine science with a passion, and suddenly, it's so much more fascinating!

Levers

Levers are handy. The smaller the lever, the easier it is for your muscles. The larger the lever, the more work you have to do, not just with pole work but with floorwork too. Also, upside down, if you're moving your body (or centre of mass) to the side, you're potentially hinged by a lever. The amount of force going into the pole from that lever point is bigger the further your body is from the pole. Thus, the more muscle stabilisation is needed.

Definition of lever[20] (Oxford Dictionary - Lexico Online. n.d)

1: a rigid bar resting on a pivot, used to move a heavy or firmly fixed load with one end when pressure is applied to the other.

Our mass in motion from earlier in this chapter isn't all that makes pole dancing, is it? We need momentum to do it. We need to move in a single direction (velocity) by using force (push/pull/swing) to move our centre of gravity. And last but not least, we need to remove contact with the ground to generate momentum.

Don't forget to then move in the other direction to even up your muscles!

Discovering the Evolution of the Warm-Up

Gone are the days when someone calls for warm-up and everyone plonks themselves on the ground. When you think of it like that, how does having a cold muscle sitting on the ground and leaning forward make that muscle warm?

Everyone knows that warm muscles have a bigger range of motion, yet we stretch cold ones. I, personally, always enjoyed stretching. It was almost relaxing, getting your brain in the zone to train, and over time, you saw increases in your flexibility.

But static stretching at the beginning of a session is now supposed to be out the door! It makes sense. I transferred my relaxing warm-ups to flowing movements, sometimes in the form of stories before increasing the tempo and getting my blood pumping. Moving through joints in a flowing manner can be just as relaxing. Warm up stories? Yes, you heard right; I work a lot with kids and take them on journeys with their movements for warm-ups, sometimes to space, or through storms, or through the ocean, there is many an adventure that can be had when you break down the movements and what creature or thing that movement can represent. My mum always said to turn work into a game, to make it fun, and a warm up should be no different.

To get technical, your body has countless mechanisms that need to be activated and stimulated in order to safely conduct rigorous physical activity. Putting your body through a series of active stretches while doing the movement you're preparing for sends signals from the brain, through the nervous system, to the muscle fibres and connective tissues in that area, telling them to prepare to do more work. Your body's temperature starts to rise, and blood is pumped to the areas of the body that are doing the work. Getting good blood flow to the muscles you want to work is critical in supplying that area with the energy it needs. This gets proper blood flow to the working area, and your muscle fibres and connective tissues will also gain more flexibility and range of motion from practising the motion.

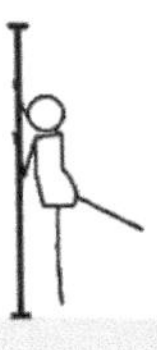

So, you need to move your muscles to warm up, but people say you need to stretch. There are multiple different types of stretching, not just static stretching.

1. Ballistic stretching, isn't seen very often, it uses the momentum of a moving body or even a limb in an attempt to force it beyond its normal range of motion. This is generally not a recommended technique.
2. Dynamic stretching involves moving parts of your body in a controlled manner and gradually increasing reach, speed of movement, or both.
3. Active stretching involves assuming a position and then holding the position with no assistance other than the strength of your agonist muscles. This means holding your leg up with your leg muscles, not your hand.
4. Passive (or relaxed) stretching is similar to active stretching, but you can use your hand, a barre, or something similar to hold the limb.
5. Static stretching involves stretching to the farthest point and holding the stretch.
6. Isometric stretching involves stretching using resistance, pushing back against something.
7. PNF stretching involves increasing static-passive flexibility by combining passive and isometric stretching. It is usually performed with a partner.

A number of research teams have tried to find out how dynamic stretching, static stretching, or no stretching affect performance. At the Department of Physical Therapy at Wichita State University, L Parsons and his research team focused on long-jump testing. At the Human Performance Laboratory at Hokkaido University, Taichi Yamaguchi and Kojiro Ishii worked on leg extension exercises. Both groups found that athletes who did dynamic stretching before exercise showed significant improvements in performance than those who did static stretching or who didn't stretch at all.

Did you know that by warming up your muscles, you're also warming up your fascia? This is also something you can specifically focus on warming up occasionally.

To put it basically, a picture of a muscle is red, and there are white bits around it and on the ends. That is your fascia. The fascinating thing about this stuff is that it's not just related to the muscles. It's everywhere. It weaves through your muscles and goes through your whole body like a spiderweb, holding everything together. Yet there isn't much out there about it.

Remember how, as a kid, you could swing your arms around everywhere, following the path of least resistance and finally just flopping over? This most likely involved moving using your fascia, not moving by only working your muscles (which, of course, moves your fascia too).

Now that the fun kid stage is gone, you do a similar thing, but it's slow and controlled. It brings you to the same folded-over end point, and you can feel it. You fatigue, and you feel your muscles working. Strange, right? Different types of movements activate different things within your body. It's still common practice to ignore fascia, but being such a massive part of your body, it affects movement and can affect mobility.

Tom Myers has done some amazing research on fascia and how it runs through the body and affects movement. Karin Gurtner, inspired by and working alongside Tom, has expanded this research into the realm of movement[21].

Ignoring fascia can dehydrate it as well as lessen its elasticity (among other things). It's not being used, so it gets less of what it needs from the body, and this can affect your mobility. Think of your fascia like your hair. If you don't care for it and brush it, it gets knotty and stiff. This is the same with every aspect of your body. Your body needs a little care but beware not to overdo it.

In saying that, your fascia is not something you want to look at stretching. That isn't how you care for it. You can awaken and vitalise your fascia by rolling to hydrate it (massage ball bliss), engaging and releasing, and all sorts of other stuff. But don't do this too often, just every few days, maybe even once a week. It's a good idea to wake up your fascia, but don't overdo it!

There you have it; things have changed. The expected thing these days is to partake in an active warm-up with dynamic stretches, not to plonk yourself on the floor to prepare for exercise. So let's get out there and get active!

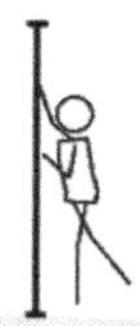

Using a Spotter

Okay, so you aren't quite there yet, but you can see the doors opening up to new and exciting moves, so let's discuss what a spotter really is.

The role of a spotter is not to hoist you up the pole. Their role is to protect your head, neck, and back. They are to have their hands up, always ready and prepared. They aren't doing the work for you; they aren't holding you on the pole.

If an instructor squeezes your thighs onto the pole or tilts your hips in a move, this isn't spotting. This is guidance so that you can feel how the move should work. This should be done by a trained professional who knows what they're doing. Once your body feels the move, you can start working on making that feeling happen without guidance.

Here's the bit you don't want to hear: if you can't get down, you shouldn't get up! The experience isn't there, and last-minute bailouts are scary! I train pre-emptive exercises and conditioning moves to deadlift into moves for many weeks before practising the position from the ground. Then I consider using momentum to help me get there. As I train to deadlift and am quite solid in conditioning drills, I know that I can safely use momentum to get into the move. That's my understanding of my body and how it works.

Don't try to do big jumps in moves. It's dangerous! When you're ready, you can glide or sweep your body in using momentum. Alternatively, keep practising until you have the strength to deadlift in. Either way, break each move down into small achievable goals. These small goals mean you can see and feel yourself getting closer without getting disheartened about not being there yet, all while keeping yourself safe.

When you go to try a big move, explain to your spotter what you're going to do. This way, they'll know where to stand so they don't get kicked and also where they should support you. A spotter is a worst-case-scenario helper, not a 'just get me up there' person. Using unqualified spotters for guidance if you aren't ready to go into a move can cause both you and your spotter injury. The idea is to prevent that, so don't rush yourself!

If you go into a hospital and ask about spinal accidents, you'll find that a vast majority happen from a height below 2 metres, as it is perceived as a safe height. Now, pole fitness is a little bit different from this, as many of the moves are perceived as impossible when you first look. Don't get me wrong, it is still high risk, and all levels of caution need to be taken. It takes a lot of training to orientate yourself with the pole, then gain grip to spin, stabilise your shoulders, and lift to climb. Then we look at partial tilts before even considering inverts. These steps protect against many incidents, coupled with the fact that the moves aren't perceived as easy, so more caution is taken. Having a spotter doesn't mean that you throw caution to the wind!

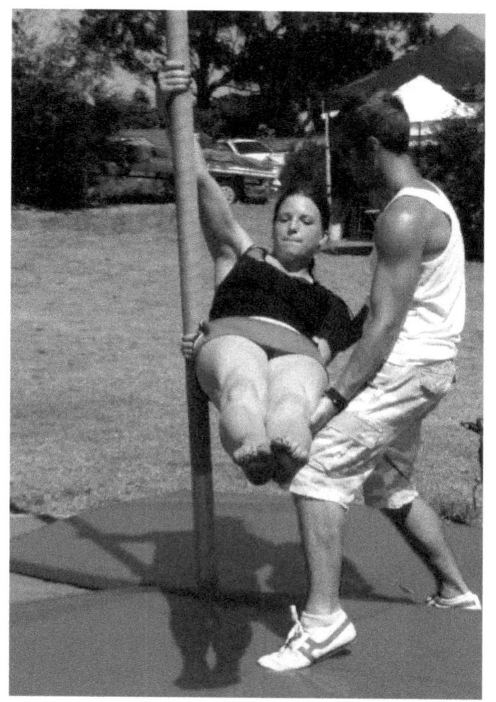

Spotters are a must. Learning new moves, you have an instructor to guide you, but beginning to do moves yourself is a whole new ball game! Having a spotter is very important. It's essential that you understand what a spotter's role is and ensure you're ready for that step.

Remember, your spotter's role is to protect your head, neck, and back. They have their hands up, always ready, and are prepared to protect your head, neck, and back while also protecting their own. If you cannot get up without a spotter holding or pushing- you are not ready for the move, and more conditioning and preparation is required. The last thing you want is 2 injured people and no one to call for help.

This also goes for crash-mats. They are not there for you to just let go and fall on. You must still control the move safely and dismount safely otherwise you are not ready for the move and need to go back to your preparation and conditioning moves. Crash-mats are a back-up that you should not rely on, you need to be able to rely on your abilities and be confident in the process otherwise you risk causing injury to yourself. Crash-mats are just a bonus, a necessary bonus, but a bonus none the less.

Tracking your Progress

One thing that helps on days when you get in a rut is to really see your progress.

At Rapture Arts, we have certificates with photos so that people have a visual record of how far they've come. It's always important to recognise and celebrate growth. That way, when you do have days that are frustrating, you can remember how far you've come.

Tracking each training session also helps you to put the little ah-ha moments on paper. Make note of things that click after weeks or months of training so that you don't suddenly forget the trick. I have post-it notes everywhere with little notes for each move. These notes include wording, positioning, and analogies that help me get moves right.

You can also write down what you want to improve on with tricks. It may be a transition into another move, a new way in or out of a move, or even a strength/flexibility goal. By writing these down, when you do have a trickier day, you can look back and find something you can work on so you still feel that sense of accomplishment.

Some people learn from doing, while others learn from seeing, listening, or writing. Working out your learning type can help you with your training.

Your physical and mental state can also play a big role in your progress. It's a great idea to make note of your fatigue and stress levels. How do you feel before training? This can affect your progress and influence what you train to prevent injury.

Need to see your goal? Create a moodboard! Where do you want to be in 6 or 12 months? Use images and colours. You can even leave spaces for photos of your progressions, adding something each month to help you stay accountable. Photo progressions are also a good tracking method for those who need to do things to learn. You could even pop a few notes next to the photos. We put in extra effort for photos to ensure that lines are right, toes are pointed, and so on. That extra attention to detail goes a long way!

Does writing work for you? I've included a, excerpt from my book, it's a training tracker called "*Personal Pole and Aerial Record*"[23]. This record notes what you're training each day, and it allows you to plan and track patterns in what works for you. There's also a self-evaluation or reflection sheet. Self-reflection is a massive thing for growth. Seeing what you did, what helped, how you grew, and where you want to go from here is important. It helps you create a clear path to achieving your goals. Reflections are great to look back on and review when needed.

The important thing is to celebrate your achievements. Celebrate trying to train on a sweltering hot day and doing a floorwork session so that you don't just skip training. Or celebrate coming out of moves smoothly, pointing your toes, or having amazing hand placement. Every little bit counts! It doesn't even have to be a move. Maybe you've been working on your lifts and can get your toes off the ground or tuck your knees to your belly. Those are massive steps. Be proud of yourself!

Date: **Level:**

Getting started *(10 min)*		
Cardio warm-up	Dynamic stretches	Conditioning

Core moves to work on today		
Move name: *(sketch if needed)*	Move name: *(sketch if needed)*	Move name: *(sketch if needed)*
Prep move 1:	Prep move 1:	Prep move 1:
Prep move 2:	Prep move 2:	Prep move 2:

Choreography notes

Cool down and stretch *(10 min)*

Self-Evaluation

Notes to improve and work on next time

Tips that helped me today		
Move name:	Move name:	Other:

Something that really clicked with me today
Favourite or inspiring music track

My goal (something I'm looking forward to)
Are you interested in the personal pole record? The Personal Pole and Aerial Record is available as a workbook for you to utilise in your training. ISBN: 978-0-6450176-2-5.

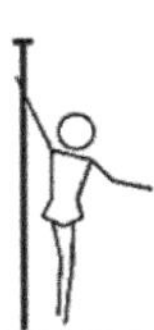

 *I'm proud of myself because …*

Moving Up the Pole

Before rushing ahead, you need to check in on your progress. Not all moves click with everyone, but it's good to see an overview and get a sense of where you're at before you move on.

Core Pole Move	I can do it on my		I can transition smoothly		Variation?
	left side	right side	into move	out of move	*(personal notes)*
Basic fireman					
Front-knee hook					
Back-knee hook					
Split grip fireman					
Windmill/fan kick					
Martini spin					
Pike spin					
Lift and slide					
One-handed fireman					
One-handed front-knee hook					
Straddle spin					
Backward spiral					
Fireman-to-pole stand					
Low-lift fireman					
Basic cradle					
Peter Pan spin					
Chair spin					
Carousel					
Basic teddy					
Side-pole slide					

Most importantly, how do you feel around the pole? How does your grip feel? Your pole journey is unique to you, and your body and movements are unique in themselves. Don't rush. Find your personal flow and style.

Check in with your body before and after training. Take note of how well you slept and where your stress levels are at. These will affect your performance. You can tally these things up and record them with your training record.

Do you have any pain? That isn't normal, and you should go and see a healthcare professional about it. What about general soreness? If you're sore, you may need to adjust your warm-up/cool-down routine to focus on specific areas of your body, or you may need to decrease the intensity of your training. You can slowly increase the intensity of your training as your strength builds and your body adjusts.

It may not be about doing the hard tricks. It may be worth adjusting the intensity of your training in some tricks to give your body more of a chance to adjust, rest, and recover.

The next stage is exciting. You can introduce things like sitting and climbing and the umpteen variations of these. You can play with new grips and eventually looking at inverting.

What are the next moves on the list to learn? I would suggest playing with sitting variations for a while. I always start these down low (from a squat position) to get accustomed to the position before lifting or doing sit moves from standing. It seems to take just over a month for people to start to desensitise their inner thighs. Desensitising one area before moving on to a new soft spot is a good idea. Otherwise, there may be a move where it's all needed, and it will be one big ouch!

After over a month (or two) of training sits, climbs, pole lifts, holding, tucks, and tuck variations, I suggest looking at training invert conditioning. This conditioning is valuable for the whole pole-journey, and will take a different amount of time for everyone. Then, when the time is right, start preparing and conditioning lying on the floor, next to the pole, so your legs and hips get an idea of what they're doing on the pole before you turn your world upside down. If that is the journey you choose.

Remember, it's good practice to train to deadlift inverts to get your strength up and to keep yourself safe. Remember safe dismounts. Come down from a basic invert position nice and controlled, like a piece of wet spaghetti (that is wrapped around the pole). Look at your belly button as you slide down to protect your head and neck… *Always* look at your belly button when you descend! Do I need to say it again?! Eventually, you can get to elaborate dismounts, but from many an inverted position, getting back to the wet-spaghetti, looking at your belly-button position should be your default dismount to ensure your own safety!

That's a whole other story. Don't rush your journey. The amount of upright poses you can play with is amazing. I have a poster full of sit variations, one-handed spins, and leaps. Then there are standing variations, cradle variations, and many more fun positions you can get yourself into, some of which even get you upside down without needing to lift!

The better your understanding of how to move your body around the pole, the easier you'll get the hang of going upside down (although I'm not saying it is easy, everyone is different!) and the safer you will be. Wrapping around the pole in different ways to get down safely won't feel as odd.

If you take a short break from pole, take a step back, and start a level lower than you were. It *should* take at least 3 to 4 weeks of regular training to get your grip strength back and to get your neural pathways all working again so you feel like you know how your body is moving on and around the pole. The longer your break, the longer it will take to get back to where you were. Take it slow, and stay safe.

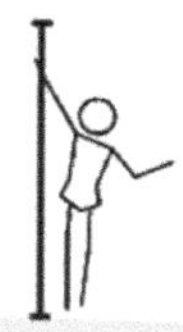

For now, enjoy the door that pole fitness has opened for you, and have fun with being able to move freely around the pole to music. Find your style, and look to your next pole goal!

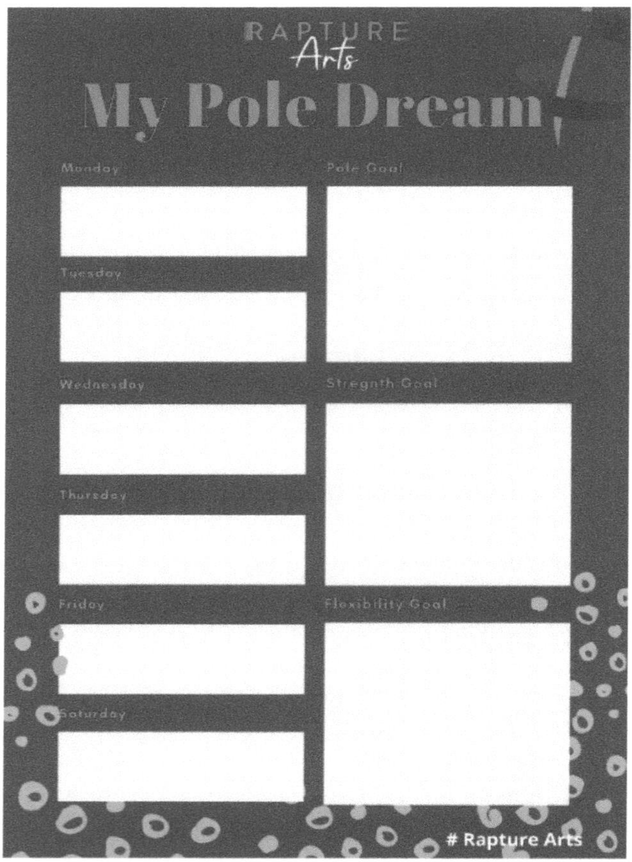

Work out what helps you train, what are your goals, what drives you and get a planner to suit your lifestyle!

My Pole Goal

MOVE GOALS

-
-
-
-
-

STEPS TO SUCCESS

STREGNTH GOALS

FLEXIBILITY GOALS

TRAINING PLAN

MONDAY	WEDNESDAY	FRIDAY

Rapture Arts

References and other sources

1. Nichols, J (2019). The psychological, physiological, and injury-related characteristics of pole dancing as a recreational activity. School of Human Sciences. doi: 10.26182/5e7d60d09e2cd. - ABC Radio Interview 'This is why women of all ages should try pole dancing – on drive with Geoff Hutchinson'

2. Adkison J, Bauer D, & Chang T (2010). The effect of topical arnica on muscle pain. *Ann Pharmacother, 44*(10), 1579-1584. doi: 10.1345/aph.1P071.

3. Knuesel O, Suter A, & Weber M (2002). Arnica montana gel in osteoarthritis of the knee: an open, multicenter clinical trial. *Adv Ther*, *19*(5), 209-218. doi: 10.1007/BF02850361.

4. Melzer J, Saller R, Suter A, & Widrig R (2007). Choosing between NSAID and arnica for topical treatment of hand osteoarthritis in a randomised, double-blind study. *Rheumatol Int., 27*(6), 585-591. doi: 10.1007/s00296-007-0304-y.

5. Ask A Medic Blog (2010, April 22). https://ucanmedic.blogspot.com/2010/04/butter-on-bruise

6. Bandy, WD & Irion, JM (1994). The effect of time on static stretch on the flexibility of the hamstring muscle. *Physical Therapy, 74*(9), 845-852. doi: 10.1093/ptj/74.9.845.

7. Wilby, N (2019). *Strength and conditioning for pole.*

8. Scherb, E (2018). *Applied anatomy of aerial arts.* North Atlantic.

9. Wiggins A (2020). *Pole sports: tracing the historical influences.*

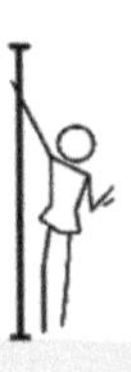

10. Brown, P J (2016, July 8). *Part II: the history and etymology of the "hoochie-coochie" dance.* Early Sports 'n' Pop-Culture History Blog.

11. Stencel A W (1999). *Girl show: into the canvas world of bump and grind.* ECW Press.

12. India Press (nd). *Sports in India.* https://sports.indiapress.org/mallakhamb.php.

13. National Geographic Society (nd). *The Silk Road.* https://www.nationalgeographic.org/encyclopedia/silk-road/.

14. Griffiths, E (2016). The history of pole dancing: a rising fitness trend. Culture Trip. https://theculturetrip.com/pacific/australia/articles/the-history-of-pole-dancing-a-rising-fitness-trend/.

15. Tatke, N & Purandare, M (2014). Enhancement of optimism as a result of participation in competitive sport – Mallakhamb. *Journal of Psychosocial Research,* *9*(1), 71-80. https://www.proquest.com/openview/54709e2ef0db09c56aa5cd0d34fba254/1?pq-origsite=gscholar&cbl=506336.

16. The Journal of Sports Medicine and Physical Fitness 2017- September; 57 (9):1098-103 - https://www.minervamedica.it/en/journals/sports-med-physical-fitness/article.php?cod=R40Y2017N09A1098

17. Grace. (2018, February 13) Chinese pole and pole dance. Similarities and differences. Gracitude. http://gracitude.com/2018/02/13/chinese-pole-vs-pole-dance/.

18. Simple English Wikipedia, the free encyclopedia. (n.d)

19. https://www.merriam-webster.com/dictionary (n.d)

20. www.lexico.com/definition/lever and https://www.encyclopedia.com/ (n.d)

21. Myers, Thomas W. Anatomy Trains: Myofascial Meridians for Manual Therapists and Movement Professionals, 4th Edition.

22. https://www.chinese-herbs.org/arnica/ (n.d.)

23. Johnson, L (2021). *Personal Pole and Aerial Record.* ISBN 978-0645017625

24. Université de Genève. "Cellular sensor of phosphate levels: Signaling molecules regulate uptake of this essential cell nutrient." ScienceDaily. ScienceDaily, 14 April 2016. <www.sciencedaily.com/releases/2016/04/160414144215.htm>.

25. R.K. Bush, S.L. Taylor, in Encyclopedia of Food Sciences and Nutrition (Second Edition), 2003

26. Tara L. Harris MD, Emalee G. Flaherty MD, in Child Abuse and Neglect, 2011 (Please note a potential trauma or emotional trigger warning reading this study. Please approach with caution.)

BONUS

BREAKDOWNS!

These are only a guide, but I hope they help you on your journey. The aim of these breakdowns is to help you prepare if you're struggling with a move. However, they do not replace professional instruction. All moves must be performed with guidance to ensure correct technique and must be paired with a balanced warm-up, dynamic stretches, and a cool-down routine.

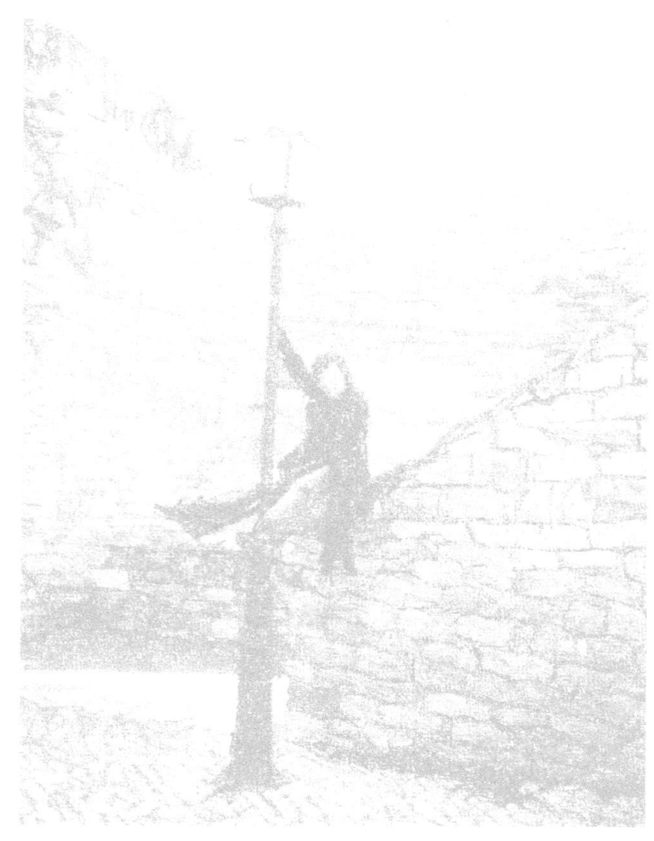

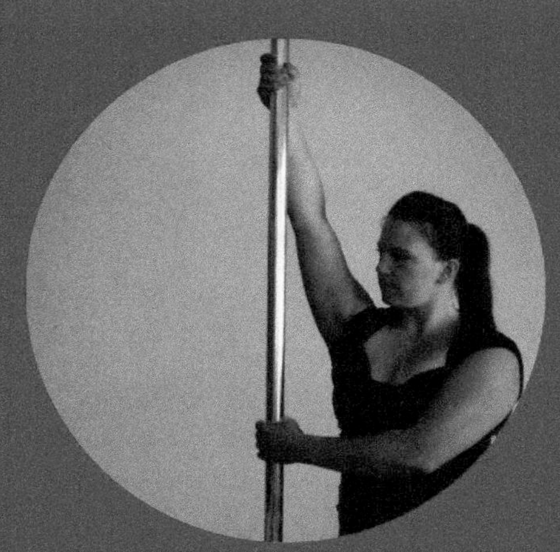

RAPTURE Arts

BASIC SPIN GRIP

Rapture Arts Adventures- Pole Move Preparation

Off the Pole

MUSCLES TO STRENGTHEN

- Shoulder Girdle and scapulae stabilisers (Trapezius, Serratus Anterior)
- Rotator Cuff (Teres Minor, Infraspinatus)
- Lower Trapezius (your wings!)

CONDITIONING

- Prone Shoulder Shrugs
- Prone Shoulder Shrugs with arm lift
- Push Ups against the wall
- Hand conditioning - finger flicks, open and close hand, spread fingers wide and together etc.

MUSCLES TO STRETCH

- Triceps
- Latissimus Dorsi
- Pectorals

STRETCHES

- Pectoral Stretches
- Shoulder stretches from all angles
- Forearm and wrist stretches

*This document is just to serve as a guide and reminder. Posture and alignment is integral. All moves must be performed under professional guidance to ensure correct technique.

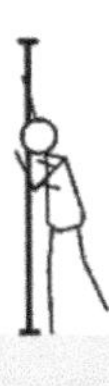

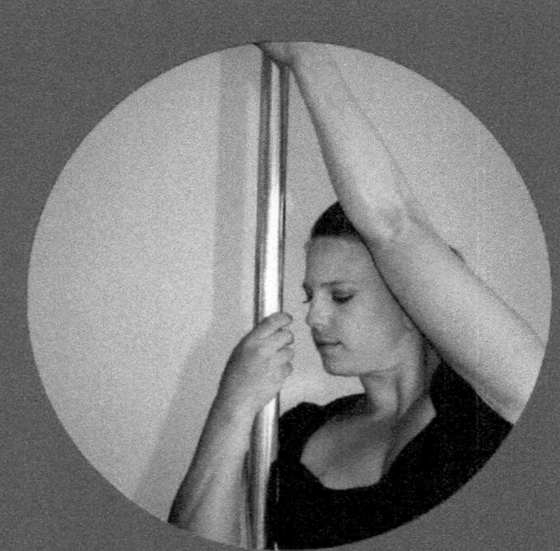

RAPTURE Arts

REVERSE SPIN GRIP

Rapture Arts Adventures- Pole Move Preparation

Off the Pole

MUSCLES TO STRENGTHEN

- Shoulder Girdle and Scapulae Stabilizers (Trapezius, Serratus Anterior)
- Rotator Cuff (Teres Minor, Infraspinatus)

CONDITIONING

- Prone Shoulder Shrugs
- Prone Shoulder Shrugs with arm lift
- Push Ups against the wall
- Hand conditioning - finger flicks, open and close hand, spread fingers wide and together etc.

MUSCLES TO STRETCH

- Triceps
- Latissimus Dorsi
- Quadratus Lumborum (side/lateral trunk flexors)

STRETCH OPTIONS

- Pectoral Stretches
- Shoulder stretches from all angles
- Forearm and wrist stretches

*This document is just to serve as a guide and reminder. Posture and alignment is integral. All moves must be performed under professional guidance to ensure correct technique.

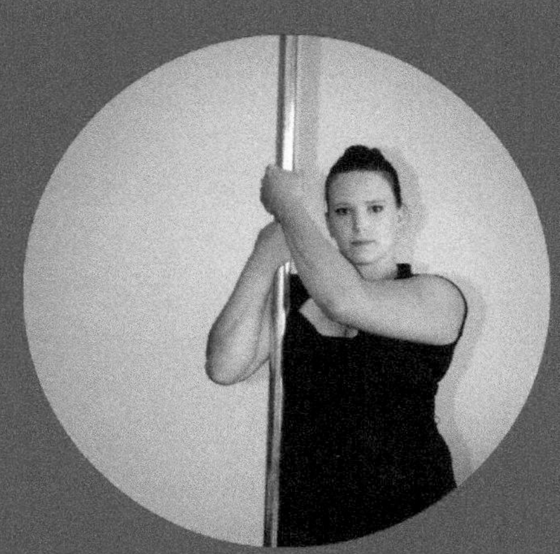

RAPTURE Arts

BASIC INVERT GRIP

Rapture Arts Adventures- Pole Move Preparation

Off the Pole

MUSCLES TO STRENGTHEN

- Shoulder Girdle and Scapulae Stabilizers (Trapezius, Serratus Anterior)
- Rotator Cuff (Teres Minor, Infraspinatus)
- Latissimus Dorsi

CONDITIONING

- Prone Shoulder Shrugs
- Prone Shoulder Shrugs with arm lift
- Push Ups against the wall
- Rowing
- Shoulder Extension
- Shoulder adduction
- Scapula setting practice

MUSCLES TO STRETCH

- Shoulder
- Pectorals
- Neck

STRETCH OPTIONS

- Pectoral Stretches
- Shoulder stretches from all angles
- Forearm and wrist stretches

*This document is just to serve as a guide and reminder. Posture and alignment is integral. All moves must be performed under professional guidance to ensure correct technique.

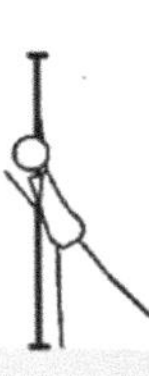

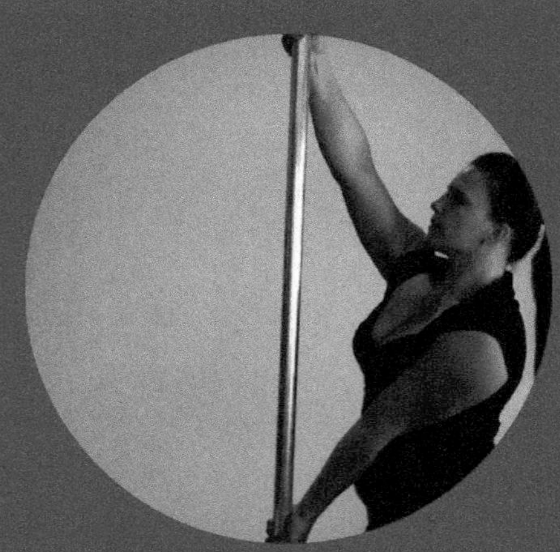

RAPTURE Arts

SPLIT GRIP

Rapture Arts Adventures- Pole Move Preparation

Off the Pole

MUSCLES TO STRENGTHEN

- Shoulder Girdle and Scapulae Stabilizers (Trapezius, Serratus Anterior) - your lower Trapezius is your wings to give you lift!
- Rotator Cuff (Teres Minor, Infraspinatus)
- Forearm Flexors
- Elbow Stabilizing muscles (if hyper extending)

CONDITIONING

- Prone Shoulder Shrugs
- Prone Shoulder Shrugs with arm lift
- Push Ups against the wall
- Hand conditioning - finger flicks, open and close hand, spread fingers wide and together etc.

CONDITIONING FOR HYPER-EXTENSION

- 4 Point kneeling-leg extension, keeping foot on ground
- 4 Point kneeling-leg extension, leg lift
- 4 Point Plank
- Prone walk outs on Fit ball (easiest is with ball at pelvis, a lttle harder at knees and hardest at feet)

MUSCLES TO STRETCH

- Triceps,
- Latissimus Dorsi
- Pectorals

STRETCH OPTIONS

- Pectoral Stretches
- Shoulder stretches from all angles
- Forearm and wrist stretches

*This document is just to serve as a guide and reminder. Posture and alignment is integral. All moves must be performed under professional guidance to ensure correct technique.

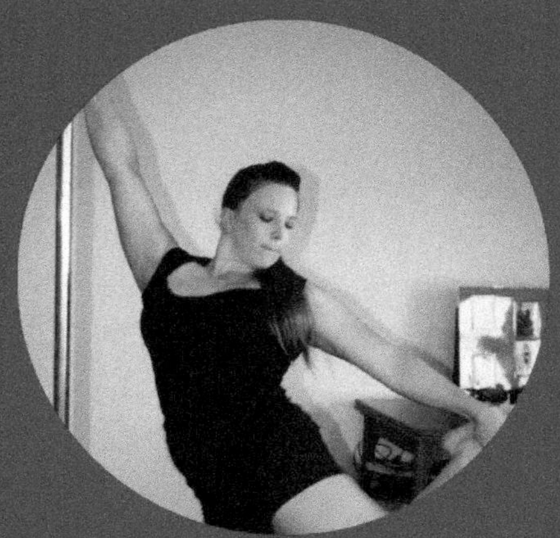

RAPTURE Arts

ONE HANDED SPINS

Rapture Arts Adventures- Pole Move Preparation

Off the Pole

MUSCLES TO STRENGTHEN

- Shoulder Girdle and Scapulae Stabilizers (Trapezius, Serratus Anterior)
- Rotator Cuff (Teres Minor, Infraspinatus)
- (Don't forget your wings- your lower Trapezius muslce)

CONDITIONING

- Prone Shoulder Shrugs
- Prone Shoulder Shrugs with arm lift
- Push Ups against the wall
- Hand conditioning - finger flicks, open and close hand, spread fingers wide and together etc.

MUSCLES TO STRETCH

- Side Flexors
- Latissimus Dorsi
- Pectorals

STRETCHES

- Pectoral Stretches
- Shoulder stretches from all angles
- Forearm and wrist stretches
- Elbow Wall slide- side on, slide arm up wall straight so whole side is touching wall.
- Vary the angle of the elbow in pec stretches, twisting body slightly

*This document is just to serve as a guide and reminder. Posture and alignment is integral. All moves must be performed under professional guidance to ensure correct technique

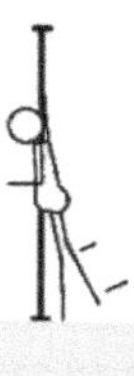

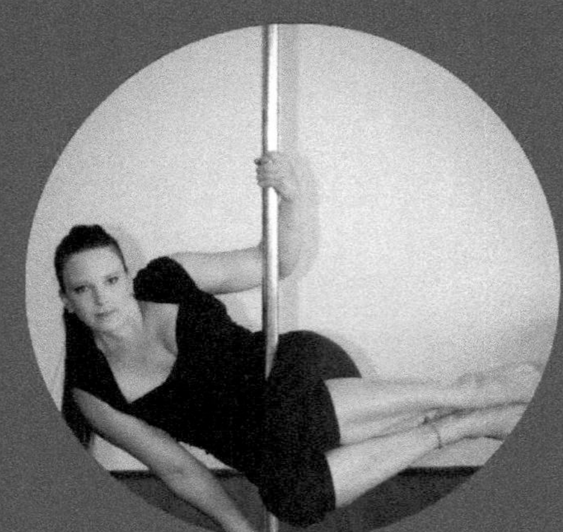

RAPTURE Arts

CRADLE GRIP

Rapture Arts Adventures- Pole Move Preparation

Off the Pole

MUSCLES TO STRENGTHEN

- Shoulder Girdle, and Scapulae Stabilizers (Trapezius, Serratus Anterior)
- Rotator Cuff (Teres Minor, Infraspinatus)
- Forearm Flexors
- Elbow Stabilizing muscles (if hyper extending)
- Biceps
- Abdominals and Obliques
- Latissimus Dorsi

CONDITIONING

- Prone Shoulder Shrugs
- Prone Shoulder Shrugs with arm lift
- Push Ups against the wall
- Bicep Curls
- Abdominal Crunches
- Abdominal Crunches with twist
- Side Plank
- Hand conditioning - finger flicks, open and close hand, spread fingers wide and together etc.

CONDITIONING FOR HYPER-EXTENSION

- 4 Point kneeling-leg extension, keeping foot on ground
- 4 Point kneeling-leg extension, leg lift
- 4 Point Plank
- Prone walk outs on Fit ball (easiest is with ball at pelvis, a little harder at knees and hardest at feet)

MUSCLES TO STRETCH

- Triceps
- Latissimus Dorsi
- Pectorals

STRETCH OPTIONS

- Pectoral Stretches
- Shoulder stretches from all angles
- Forearm and wrist stretches

*This document is just to serve as a guide and reminder. Posture and alignment is integral. All moves must be performed under professional guidance to ensure correct technique.

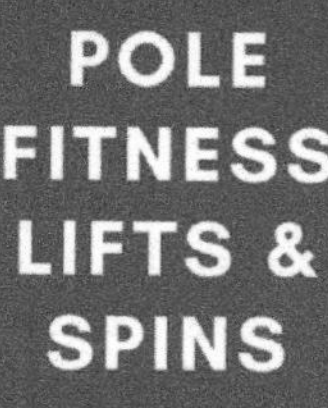
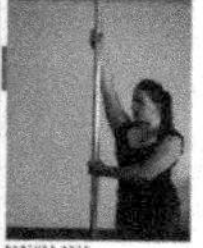
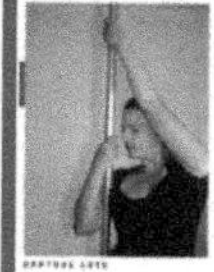
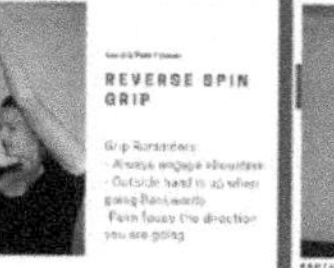
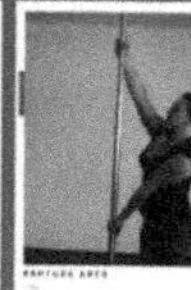
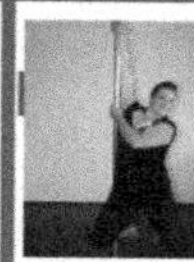
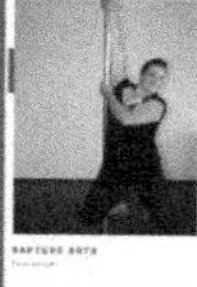
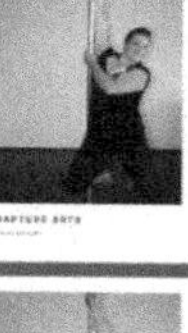
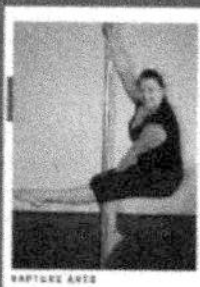
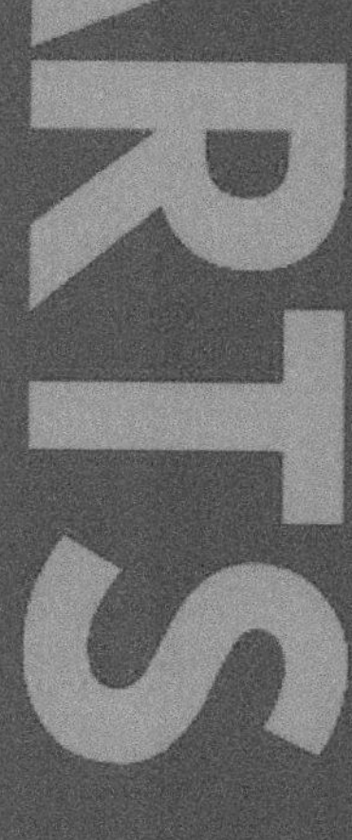
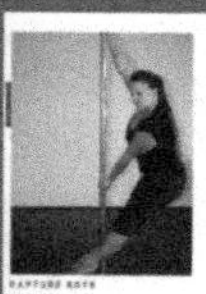
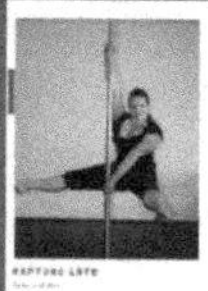
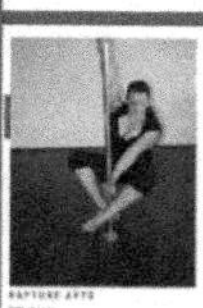
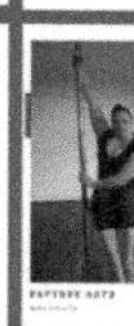
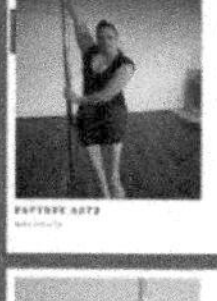
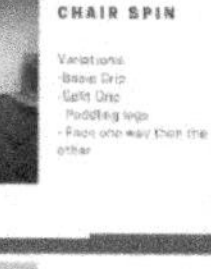

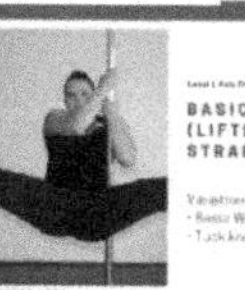
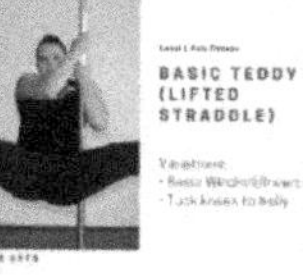
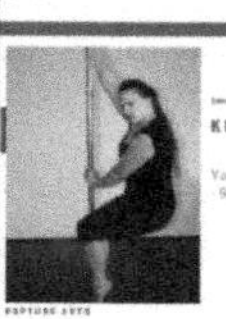
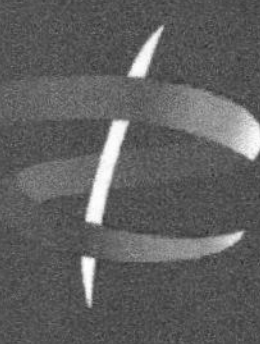
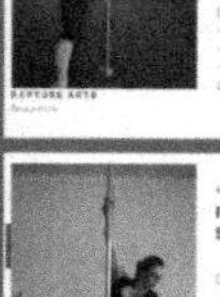
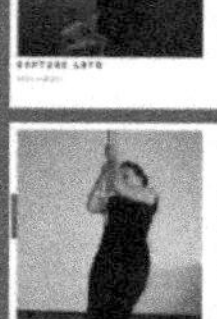
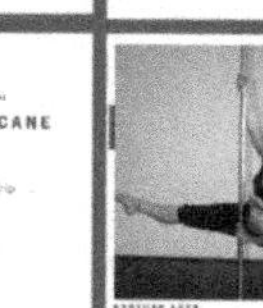
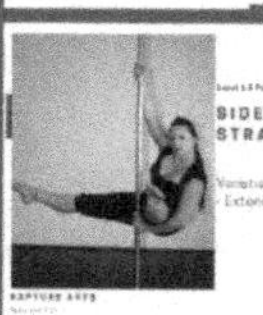
POLE FITNESS LIFTS & SPINS
RAPTURE
ARTS
BASIC GRIP
REVERSE SPIN GRIP
SPLIT GRIP
WINDMILL/ BASIC INVERT GRIP
FIREMAN SPIN
FORWARDS KNEES
BACKWARDS KNEES
WINDMILL
MARTINI SPIN
PIKE SPIN
STRADDLE SPIN
LIFT AND SLIDE
BACKWARDS SPIRAL
FIREMAN TO STAND
LOW LIFT SPIN
BASIC CRADLE
PETER PAN
CHAIR SPIN
CAROUSEL
SWAN
BASIC TEDDY (LIFTED STRADDLE)
POLE SLIDE
DOUBLE FORWARD KNEES
KNEE HUG
FIREMAN KICK SPIN
CANDY CANE
SIDE STRADDLE
LEVEL 1 & 1.5

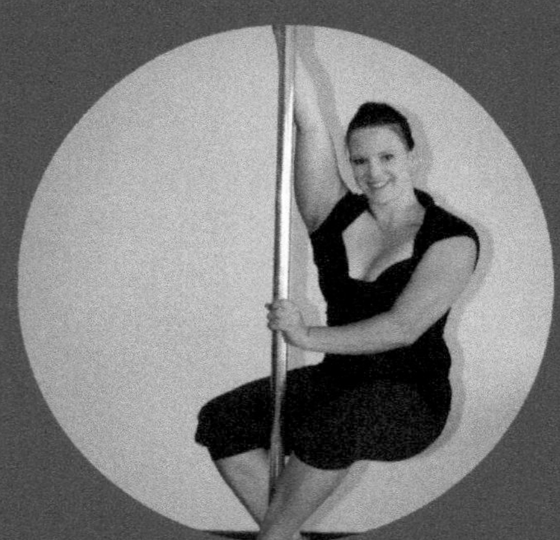

RAPTURE Arts

FIREMAN SPIN

Rapture Arts Adventures- Pole Move Preparation

Off the Pole

MUSCLES TO STRENGTHEN

- Hip flexors
- Shoulder girdle and Scapulae Stabilisers (Trapezius, Serratus Anterior)
- Rotator Cuff (Teres Minor, Infraspinatus)
- Pelvic Floor
- All core (Abdominals and Spine)

CONDITIONING

- Prone Shoulder Shrugs
- Prone Shoulder Shrugs with arm lift
- Push Ups against the wall
- Sit up variations

GRIP CONDITIONING

- Hand conditioning - finger flicks, open and close hand, spread fingers wide and together etc.

MUSCLES TO STRETCH

- Glutes
- Hamstrings
- Triceps
- Latissimus Dorsi
- Pectorals

STRETCH OPTIONS

- Glute stretch (laying down figure 4)
- Standing Hamstring stretch
- Bilateral seated forward bend (pike stretch)
- All grip arm/chest/back/shoulder/neck stretches as per normal warm up and safe practice

*This document is just to serve as a guide and reminder. Posture and alignment is integral. All moves must be performed under professional guidance to ensure correct technique.

RAPTURE Arts

FIREMAN SPIN

Rapture Arts Adventures- Pole Move Breakdown

MUSCLES TO STRENGTHEN

- Hip flexors
- All of your core muscles
- Shoulder girdle and Scapulae stabilizers (Trapezius, Serratus Anterior)
- Rotator Cuff (Teres Minor, Infraspinatus)

MUSCLES TO STRETCH

- Glutes
- Hamstrings
- Triceps
- Latissimus Dorsi
- Pectorals

WARNING

- Ensure you roll your shoulders back and don't hang out of your joint - keep muscles engaged.
- Step into moves- jumping in them uses the force of gravity against you- you come down faster and are more likely to bruise from banging the pole

STEPS

Step 1: Inside hand up on the pole, with your elbow straight, palm facing the direction that you are going... roll the shoulder back to set your shoulder blades.

Step 2: Put your outside hand across your body, holding on at waist height.

Step 3: Step on your inside leg to bring your outside leg in front of the pole (knee on one side, ankle on the other, all of the skin of the calf touching the pole).

Step 4: Tap your other leg to the back of the pole (knee on one side, ankle on the other so that one knee is on each side of the pole with the shin against the pole).

... Spin!

REGRESSIONS

- Pole lifts, standing or on knees, lifting body onto tippy toes
- Outside hand can come higher if cant grip across chest- but do not hang out of shoulders
- False Step Arounds

PROGRESSIONS

- Play with momentum- walk into it...
- Experiment with smooth dismounts
- Split Grip Fireman
- 1 handed Fireman

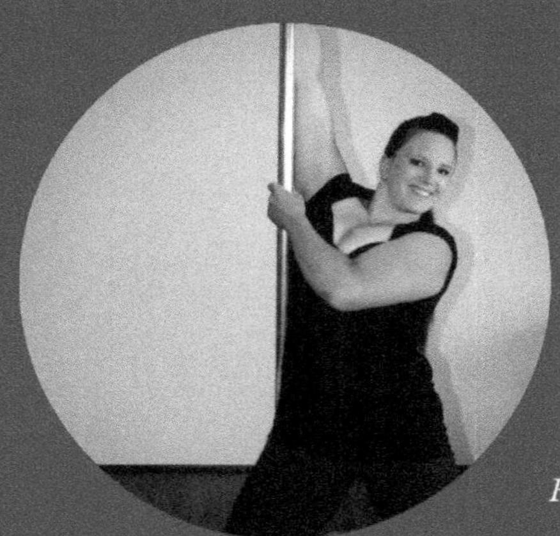

RAPTURE Arts

FRONT KNEE HOOK SPIN

Rapture Arts Adventures- Pole Move Preparation

Off the Pole

MUSCLES TO STRENGTHEN

- Hamstrings
- Shoulder girdle and scapula stabilisers (Trapezius, Serratus Anterior)
- Rotator Cuff (Teres Minor, Infraspinatus)
- Pectorals

CONDITIONING

- Prone Hamstring Curls

GRIP CONDITIONING

- Prone Shoulder Shrugs
- Prone Shoulder Shrugs with arm lift
- Push Ups against the wall
- Hand conditioning - finger flicks, open and close hand, spread fingers wide and together etc.

MUSCLES TO STRETCH

- Hip flexors
- Quads
- Triceps
- Latissimus Dorsi

STRETCH OPTIONS

- Quadriceps stretch (standing or side lying knee bend)
- Kneeling Hip Flexor Stretch (raise same arm as back leg to point to sky)
- All grip arm/chest/back/shoulder/neck stretches as per normal warm up and safe practice

*This document is just to serve as a guide and reminder. Posture and alignment is integral. All moves must be performed under professional guidance to ensure correct technique.

RAPTURE Arts

FRONT KNEE HOOK SPIN

Rapture Arts Adventures- Pole Move Breakdown

MUSCLES TO STRENGTHEN

- Hamstrings
- Shoulder girdle and scapula stabilisers (Trapezius, Serratus Anterior)
- Rotator Cuff (Teres Minor, Infraspinatus)
- Pectorals

MUSCLES TO STRETCH

- Hip flexors
- Quads
- Triceps
- Latissimus Dorsi

WARNING

- Ensure you roll your shoulders back and don't hang out of your joint, keep muscles engaged.
- Step into moves- jumping in them uses the force of gravity against you- you come down faster and are more likely to bruise from banging the pole.

STEPS

Step 1: Inside hand up on the pole, palm facing the direction you are going... roll the shoulder back;

Step 2: Outside hand across body holding on at chest height;

Step 3: Bend your inside leg onto the pole at a comfortable, natural height.

Step 4: Up onto the ball of your outside foot

Step 5: Lean forwards through the hips, as if falling; bending the outside leg when it needs to- let gravity do the work!

Spin! To the floor! (going to the floor means 2 extra seconds of conditioning)

REGRESSIONS

- Pole lifts, standing or on knees, lifting body onto tippy toes
- Outside hand can come higher if cant grip across chest- but do not hang out of shoulders

PROGRESSIONS

- Play with momentum- walk into it...
- Experiment with smooth dismounts
- Front knee hook to both knees in front of pole
- 1 handed Forwards Knees/Front Knee hook
- Forwards Knees into backwards knees

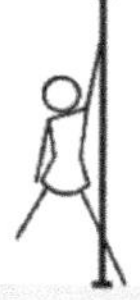

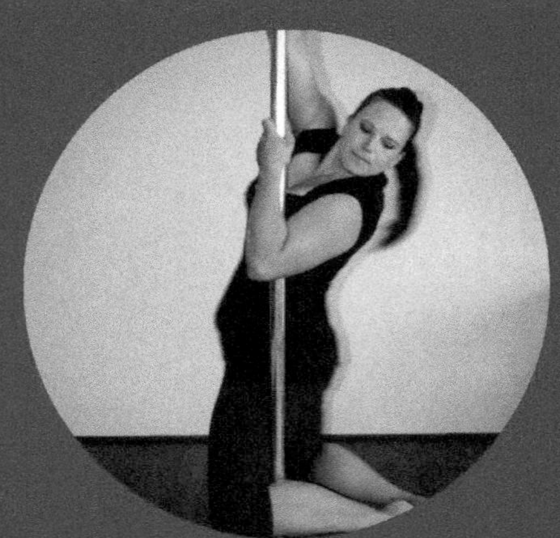

RAPTURE Arts

BACK KNEE HOOK SPIN

Rapture Arts Adventures- Pole Move Preparation

Off the Pole

MUSCLES TO STRENGTHEN

- Hamstrings
- Shoulder girdle and shoulder stabilisers (Trapezius, Serratus Anterior)
- Rotator Cuff (Teres Minor, Infraspinatus)
- Pectorals

CONDITIONING

- Straight leg raises (standing)

GRIP CONDITIONING

- Prone Shoulder Shrugs
- Prone Shoulder Shrugs with arm lift
- Push Ups against the wall
- Hand conditioning - finger flicks, open and close hand, spread fingers wide and together etc.

MUSCLES TO STRETCH

- Hip flexors
- Quads
- Triceps
- Latissimus Dorsi
- Quadratus Lumborum (side/lateral trunk flexors)

STRETCH OPTIONS

- Quadriceps stretch (standing or side lying knee bend)
- Kneeling Hip Flexor Stretch (raise same arm as back leg to point to sky)
- All grip arm/chest/back/shoulder/neck stretches as per normal warm up and safe practice

*This document is just to serve as a guide and reminder. Posture and alignment is integral. All moves must be performed under professional guidance to ensure correct technique.

RAPTURE Arts

BACK KNEE HOOK SPIN

Rapture Arts Adventures- Pole Move Breakdown

MUSCLES TO STRENGTHEN

- Hamstrings
- Shoulder girdle and shoulder stabilisers (Trapezius, Serratus Anterior)
- Rotator Cuff (Teres Minor, Infraspinatus)
- Pectorals

MUSCLES TO STRETCH

- Hip flexors
- Quads
- Triceps
- Latissimus Dorsi
- Quadratus Lumborum (side/lateral trunk flexors)

WARNING

- Ensure you roll your shoulders back and dont hang out of your joint.
- Step into moves- jumping in them uses the force of gravity against you- you come down faster and are more likely to bruise from banging the pole.

STEPS

Step 1: Roll your shoulder back... Outside hand up, palm facing the direction you are going (behind you);

Step 2: Inside hand wraps around the pole at shoulder height;

Step 3: Inside foot on its toe in front of the pole- give it a wag to make sure you don't hit the pole.

Step 4: Transfer your weight onto the inside foot (ball of the foot)

Step 5: Draw a circle starting in front, going behind you with your outside leg

Step 6: As your inside calf touches, bend your knees.... Spin! (using gravity) ... To the floor! (going to the floor means 2 extra seconds of conditioning)

REGRESSIONS

- Pole lifts, standing or on knees, lifting body onto tippy toes.
- Outside hand can come higher if cant grip across chest- but do not hang out of shoulders.

PROGRESSIONS

- Play with momentum- walk into it...
- Experiment with smooth dismounts
- Forwards Knees into Backwards Knees
- Pirouette or False Step around into Backwards Knees/Back Knee hook

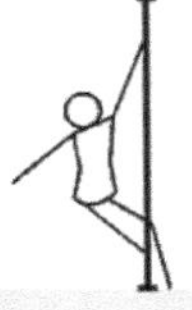

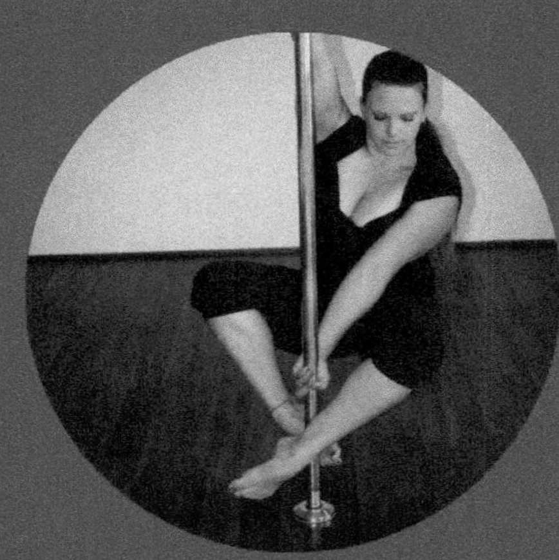

RAPTURE Arts

SPLIT GRIP FIREMAN SPIN

Rapture Arts Adventures- Pole Move Preparation

Off the Pole

MUSCLES TO STRENGTHEN

- Hip flexors
- Shoulder girdle and Scapulae Stabilizers (Trapezius, Serratus Anterior)
- Abdominals, (All core- including spine)
- Pelvic Floor
- Forearm flexors
- Elbow stability muscles (if hyper extensive in the elbows)

CONDITIONING

- Front Plank on elbows and knees
- Side Plank on elbows and knees
- Standing hip flexion with resistance band

GRIP CONDITIONING

- Prone Shoulder Shrugs
- Prone Shoulder Shrugs with arm lift
- Push Ups against the wall
- Potential conditioning to stop hyper extension of the elbow
- Hand conditioning - finger flicks, open and close hand, spread fingers wide and together etc.

MUSCLES TO STRETCH

- Glutes
- Adductors
- Hip Flexors

STRETCH OPTIONS

- Glute stretch (laying down figure 4)
- Pigeon Pose
- Butterfly (groin stretch)
- 1/2 Straddle Stretches (one leg bent in)
- Kneeling hip flexor stretch (same arm as back leg up)
- All grip arm/chest/back/shoulder/neck stretches as per normal warm up and safe practice

*This document is just to serve as a guide and reminder. Posture and alignment is integral. All moves must be performed under professional guidance to ensure correct technique.

RAPTURE
Arts

SPLIT GRIP FIREMAN SPIN

Rapture Arts Adventures- Pole Move Breakdown

MUSCLES TO STRENGTHEN

- Hip flexors
- Shoulder girdle and Scapulae stabilisers (Trapezius, Serratus Anterior)
- Abdominals (and the rest of the core),
- Forearm flexors
- Elbow stability muscles (if hyper extensive in the elbows)

MUSCLES TO STRETCH

- Glutes
- Adductors
- Hip Flexors

WARNING

- Ensure you roll your shoulders back and don't hang out of your joint
- Actively pull with your top arm or you will get a pain in your lower forearm
- Place limbs onto pole to avoid bruising
- Step into moves-not jump

*Guide Only: does not replace professional training or tuition

STEPS

Step 1: Roll your shoulder back... Inside hand up, palm facing the direction you are going;
Step 2: Step on your inside leg and pivot to face the pole
Step 3: Place your outside hand on the pole, with your finger pointing down the pole
Step 4: Bring your outside leg around, in front of pole tapping your ankle onto the pole .... Pull with your top arm, push with your bottom arm...
Step 5: Tap the other leg to the back of the pole ... Spin!

REGRESSIONS

- Pole lifts, standing or on knees, lifting body onto tippy toes
- Shoulder Shrug lifts
- Laying Shoulder Squeezes
- Basic Fireman

PROGRESSIONS

- Play with momentum- walk into it...
- Experiment with smooth dismounts
- 1 handed Fireman
- Martini

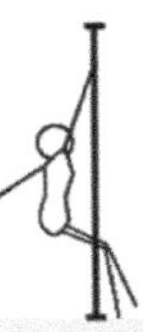

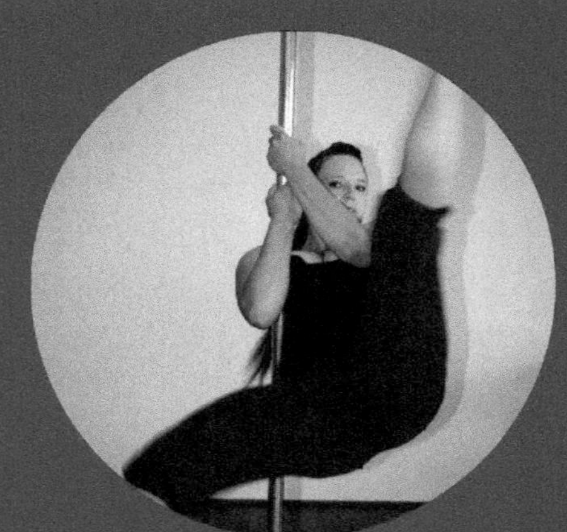

RAPTURE Arts

WINDMILL

Rapture Arts Adventures- Pole Move Preparation

Off the Pole

MUSCLES TO STRENGTHEN

- Hip Flexors
- Shoulder girdle and Scapulae Stabilizers (Trapezius, Serratus Anterior)
- Rotator Cuff (Teres Minor, Infraspinatus)
- Abdominals
- Latissimus Dorsi

CONDITIONING

- Abdominal Crunch
- Side Plank with arm peel (top arm under torso and open to sky) *can be on your elbow
- Standing Hip Flexion- with resistance band

GRIP CONDITIONING

- Prone Shoulder Shrugs
- Prone Shoulder Shrugs with arm lift
- Push Ups against the wall
- Rowing
- Shoulder Extension
- Shoulder adduction
- Scapula setting practice
- Hand conditioning - finger flicks, open and close hand, spread fingers wide and together etc.

MUSCLES TO STRETCH

- Glutes
- Hamstrings

STRETCH OPTIONS

- Standing Hamstring stretch
- Bilateral seated forward bend (pike stretch)
- Glute stretch (laying down figure 4)
- Lying- down pretzel stretch
- All grip arm/chest/back/shoulder/neck stretches as per normal warm up and safe practice

RAPTURE Arts

WINDMILL

Rapture Arts Adventures- Pole Move Breakdown

MUSCLES TO STRENGTHEN

- Hip Flexors
- Shoulder girdle and Scapulae stabilisers (Trapezius, Serratus Anterior)
- Rotator Cuff (Teres Minor, Infraspinatus)
- Abdominals (and core muscles),
- Latissimus Dorsi.

MUSCLES TO STRETCH

- Glutes
- Hamstrings

WARNING

- Ensure you roll your shoulders back and don't hang out of your joint., keep your muscles engaged. Actively pull with your top arm or you will get a pain in your lower forearm
- Place limbs onto pole to avoid bruising
- Step into moves-not jump.

STEPS

Step 1: Inside arm comes around the pole holding the pole at face height, elbow down

Step 2: Outside hand also at face height

Step 3: Squeeze your inside arm onto the pole

Step 4: Take a small step with your outside leg, so that you can kick your inside leg- away from the pole (hip in front if pole)

Step 5: Circle it around (draw your rainbow) – the other leg should then follow

Step 6: pivot to face pole

REGRESSIONS

- Pole lifts, standing or on knees, lifting on to toes
- Basic grip Fireman
- Forward Knee Hook
- Back Knee Hook
- Windmill on the ground

PROGRESSIONS

- Experiment with pivot turns, and other flow on moves.

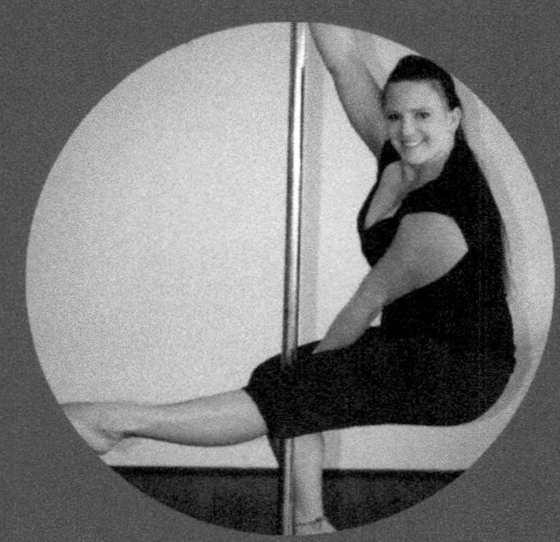

RAPTURE Arts

MARTINI SPIN

Rapture Arts Adventures- Pole Move Preparation

Off the Pole

MUSCLES TO STRENGTHEN

- Hip flexors
- Shoulder girdle and Scapulae Stabilizers (Trapezius, Serratus Anterior)
- Pelvic Floor
- All core (Abdominals and Spine)
- Abductors
- Forearm flexors
- Elbow stability muscles (if hyper extensive in the elbows)

CONDITIONING

- Ball between knees- wall squats
- Hip flexion in standing with resistance band
- straight leg raise- standing with resistance band

GRIP CONDITIONING

- Prone Shoulder Shrugs
- Prone Shoulder Shrugs with arm lift
- Push Ups against the wall
- Potential conditioning to stop hyper extension of the elbow
- Hand conditioning - finger flicks, open and close hand, spread fingers wide and together etc.

MUSCLES TO STRETCH

- Glutes,
- Hamstrings

STRETCH OPTIONS

- Standing Hamstring stretch
- Bilateral seated forward bend (pike stretch)
- All grip arm/chest/back/shoulder/neck stretches as per normal warm up and safe practice

*This document is just to serve as a guide and reminder. Posture and alignment is integral. All moves must be performed under professional guidance to ensure correct technique.

RAPTURE Arts

MARTINI SPIN

Rapture Arts Adventures- Pole Move Breakdown

MUSCLES TO STRENGTHEN

- Hip flexors
- Shoulder girdle and Scapulae stabilisers (Trapezius, Serratus Anterior)
- Abdominals (and the rest of the core),
- Adductors
- Forearm flexors
- Elbow stability muscles (if hyper extensive in the elbows)

MUSCLES TO STRETCH

- Glutes
- Hamstrings

WARNING

- Ensure you roll your shoulders back and don't hang out of your joint.
- Actively pull with your top arm or you will get a pain in your lower forearm
- Place limbs on to pole to avoid bruising
- Step into moves-not jump.

STEPS

Step 1: Roll your shoulder back... Inside hand up, palm facing the direction you are going;
Step 2: Step on your inside leg and pivot to face the pole.
Step 3: Place your outside hand on the pole, with your finger pointing down the pole.
Step 4: Bring your outside leg around, in front of pole keeping it straight..... Pull with your top arm, push with your bottom arm...
Step 5: The other leg sits next to the pole on the other side, or toes tucked under your bottom.

REGRESSIONS

- Pole lifts, standing or on knees, lifting body on to tippy toes
- Shoulder Shrug lifts
- Laying Shoulder Squeezes
- Split Grip Fireman

PROGRESSIONS

- Play with momentum- walk into it...
- Experiment with smooth dismounts
- Pike Spin

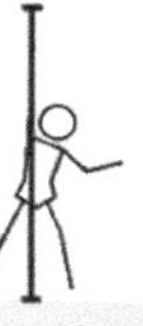

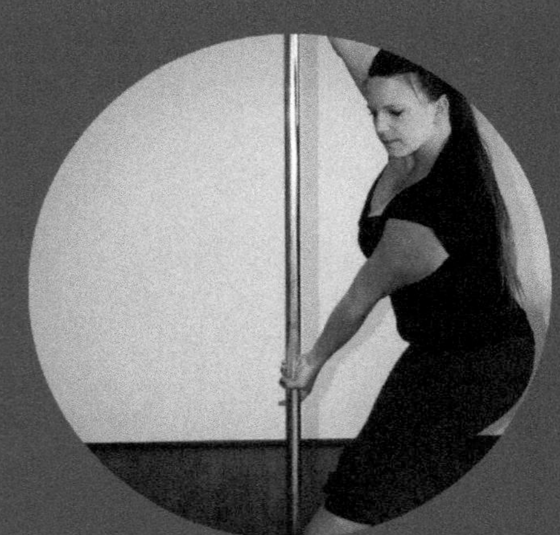

RAPTURE *Arts*

PIKE SPIN

Rapture Arts Adventures- Pole Move Preparation

Off the Pole

MUSCLES TO STRENGTHEN

- Quadriceps
- Shoulder girdle and Scapulae stability (Trapezius, Serratus Anterior)
- Pelvic Floor
- All core (Abdominals and Spine)
- Adductors
- Forearm flexors
- Elbow stability muscles (if hyper extensive in the elbows)

CONDITIONING

- Quadriceps- Squats
- Adductors- standing with resistance band

GRIP CONDITIONING

- Prone Shoulder Shrugs
- Prone Shoulder Shrugs with arm lift
- Push Ups against the wall
- Potential conditioning to stop hyper extension of the elbow
- Hand conditioning - finger flicks, open and close hand, spread fingers wide and together etc.

MUSCLES TO STRETCH

- Glutes,
- Hamstrings
- Lower Back/Lumbar

STRETCH OPTIONS

- Spinal Roll downs
- Glute stretch (laying down figure 4)
- Standing Hamstring stretch
- Bilateral seated forward bend (pike stretch)
- All grip arm/chest/back/shoulder/neck stretches as per normal warm up and safe practice

*This document is just to serve as a guide and reminder. Posture and alignment is integral. All moves must be performed under professional guidance to ensure correct technique.

RAPTURE Arts

PIKE SPIN

Rapture Arts Adventures- Pole Move Breakdown

MUSCLES TO STRENGTHEN

- Quadriceps
- Shoulder girdle and Scapulae stabilisers (Trapezius, Serratus Anterior)
- Abdominals (and the rest of the core)
- Adductors
- Forearm flexors
- Elbow stability muscles (if hyper extensive in the elbows)

MUSCLES TO STRETCH

- Glutes
- Hamstrings
- Lower Back/Lumbar

WARNING

- Ensure you roll your shoulders back and don't hang out of your joint.
- Actively pull with your top arm or you will get a pain in your lower forearm
- Place limbs on to pole to avoid bruising
- Step into moves-not jump.

STEPS

Step 1: Roll your shoulder back... Inside hand up, palm facing the direction you are going
Step 2: Step on your inside leg and pivot to face the pole.
Step 3: Place your outside hand on the pole, with your finger pointing down the pole.
Step 4: Bring your outside leg around, in front of pole keeping it straight.... Pull with your top arm, push with your bottom arm...
Step 5: The other leg pushes off the ground and comes next to it, ankles together

REGRESSIONS

- Pole lifts, standing or on knees, lifting body off ground if possible
- Shoulder Shrug lifts
- Laying Shoulder Squeezes
- Split Grip Fireman
- Martini Spin

PROGRESSIONS

- Play with momentum- walk into it...
- Experiment with smooth dismounts
- Straddle Spin

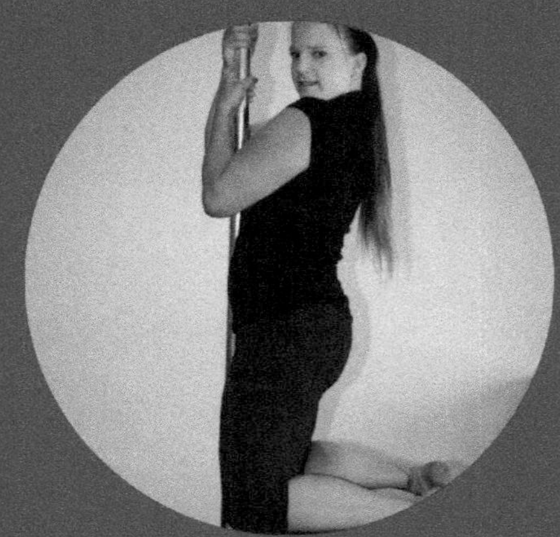

RAPTURE Arts

LIFT AND SLIDE

Rapture Arts Adventures- Pole Move Preparation

Off the Pole

MUSCLES TO STRENGTHEN

- Latissimus Dorsi
- Forearm flexors
- Bicep
- Shoulder girdle and Scapulae Stabilizers (Trapezius, Serratus Anterior)
- Rotator Cuff (Teres Minor, Infraspinatus)

CONDITIONING

- Shoulder Adduction
- Scapula Stability (set and maintain settling)
- Bicep Curls
- Forearm strength - hold a stick with some string hanging off it with two hands- roll the stick until the string is all the way rolled up the stick
- Hand conditioning - finger flicks, open and close hand, spread fingers wide and together etc.

MUSCLES TO STRETCH

- Quadriceps
- Hip Flexors

STRETCH OPTIONS

- Quadriceps stretch (standing or side lying knee bend)
- Bridging (shoulder bridge- feet and knees together)
- Kneeling Hip Flexor Stretch (raise same arm as back leg to point to sky)
- All grip arm/chest/back/shoulder/neck stretches as per normal warm up and safe practice

*This document is just to serve as a guide and reminder. Posture and alignment is integral. All moves must be performed under professional guidance to ensure correct technique.

RAPTURE Arts

LIFT AND SLIDE

Rapture Arts Adventures- Pole Move Breakdown

MUSCLES TO STRENGTHEN

- Latissimus Dorsi
- Forearm flexors
- Bicep
- Shoulder girdle and Scapulae stabilisers (Trapezius, Serratus Anterior)

MUSCLES TO STRETCH

- Quadriceps
- Hip Flexors

WARNING

- Ensure you roll your shoulders back and don't hang out of your joint, keep your muscles engaged.
- Actively pull with your top arm or you will get a pain in your lower forearm
- Place limbs on to pole to avoid bruising
- Step into moves-not jump

STEPS

Step 1: Any arm on the pole just above head height, Shoulders rolled back

Step 2: Other hand, just below the first

Step 3: Remove your feet from the floor (you want to try and keep your arms bent, and hands around face height, but this comes with time and practice)

Step 4: Slide to a kneeling position

REGRESSIONS

- Pole lifts, standing or on knees, lifting body off ground if possible
- Tuck knees onto pole to have extra grip
- Hands at face height instead of lifting up to them
- Fireman
- Forwards Knee Hook
- Back Knee Hook

PROGRESSIONS

- Play with momentum- walk into it...
- Experiment with smooth dismounts
- Lift and hold
- Lift and slow lower
- Hips in front of pole, pole lifts and tucks and hold

*Guide Only- does not replace professional training or tuition

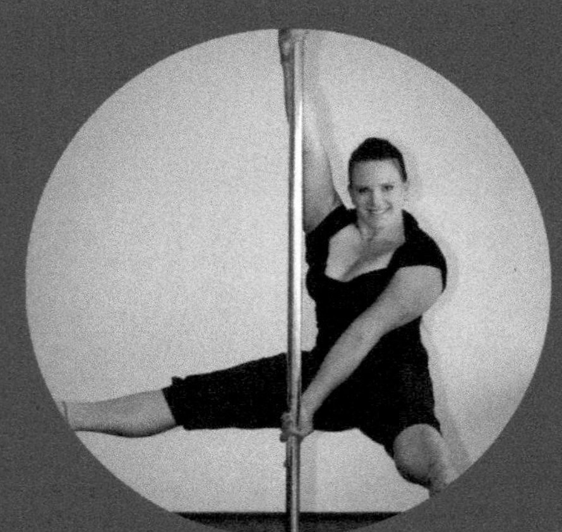

RAPTURE Arts

STRADDLE SPIN

Rapture Arts Adventures- Pole Move Preparation

Off the Pole

MUSCLES TO STREGNTHEN

- Hip Flexors
- Shoulder girdle and Scapulae Stabilizers (Trapezius, Serratus Anterior)
- Pelvic Floor
- All core (Abdominals and Spine)
- Forearm flexors
- Elbow stability muscles (if hyper extensive in the elbows)

CONDITIONING

- Front Plank
- Standing hip and knee flexion- with resistance band

GRIP CONDITIONING

- Prone Shoulder Shrugs
- Prone Shoulder Shrugs with arm lift
- Push Ups against the wall
- Potential conditioning to stop hyper extension of the elbow
- Hand conditioning - finger flicks, open and close hand, spread fingers wide and together etc.

MUSCLES TO STRETCH

- Glutes
- Hamstrings
- Lower Back/Lumbar

STRETCH OPTIONS

- Spinal Roll Downs
- Seated Straddle Stretches
- All grip arm/chest/back/shoulder/neck stretches as per normal warm up and safe practice

*This document is just to serve as a guide and reminder. Posture and alignment is integral. All moves must be performed under professional guidance to ensure correct technique.

RAPTURE Arts

STRADDLE SPIN

Rapture Arts Adventures- Pole Move Breakdown

MUSCLES TO STRENGTHEN

- Hip Flexors and Quadriceps
- Shoulder girdle and Scapulae stabilisers (Trapezius, Serratus Anterior)
- Abdominals (and the rest of the core),
- Forearm flexors
- Elbow stability muscles (if hyper extensive in the elbows)

MUSCLES TO STRETCH

- Glutes,
- Hamstrings
- Lower Back/Lumbar

WARNING

- Ensure you roll your shoulders back and don't hang out of your joint.
- Actively pull with your top arm or you will get a pain in your lower forearm,
- Place limbs onto pole to avoid bruising,
- Step into moves-not jump.

*Guide Only- does not replace professional training or tuition

STEPS

Step 1: Roll your shoulder back... Inside hand up, palm facing the direction you are going

Step 2: Step on your inside leg and pivot to face the pole

Step 3: Place your outside hand on the pole, with your finger pointing down the pole.

Step 4: Bring your outside leg up and around, stopping before you get to the pole

.... Pull with your top arm, push with your bottom arm...

Step 5: Push off the inside leg as you bring it up to spin

REGRESSIONS

- Pole lifts, standing or on knees, lifting body off ground if possible
- Shoulder Shrug lifts
- Split Grip Fireman
- Martini Spin
- Pike Spin

PROGRESSIONS

- Play with momentum- walk into it...
- Experiment with smooth dismounts.
- Straddle Spin hip circles

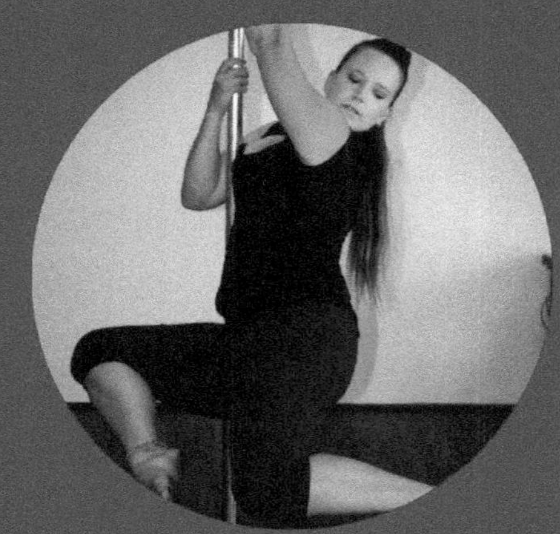

RAPTURE Arts

BACKWARDS SPRIAL

Rapture Arts Adventures- Pole Move Preparation

Off the Pole

MUSCLES TO STRENGTHEN

- Glute Med
- Abductors
- Trunk control (abs, obliques etc.)
- Shoulder girdle and Scapulae Stabilizers (Trapezius, Serratus Anterior)
- Rotator Cuff (Teres Minor, Infraspinatus)
- Pelvic Floor
- All core (Abdominals and Spine).

CONDITIONING

- Modified Clam
- Standing hip abduction with resistance band (bringing your leg away from you, and controlling it coming in)
- Plank
- Side Plank
- Side plank with leg lift

GRIP CONDITIONING

- Prone Shoulder Shrugs
- Prone Shoulder Shrugs with arm lift
- Push Ups against the wall
- Hand conditioning - finger flicks, open and close hand, spread fingers wide and together etc.

MUSCLES TO STRETCH

- Hip Flexors
- Side (obliques)
- Hip adductors

STRETCH OPTIONS

- Kneeling Hip Flexor Stretch (raise same arm as back leg to point to sky)
- All grip arm/chest/back/shoulder/neck stretches as per normal warm up and safe practice

*This document is just to serve as a guide and reminder. Posture and alignment is integral. All moves must be performed under professional guidance to ensure correct technique.

RAPTURE Arts

BACKWARDS SPRIAL

Rapture Arts Adventures- Pole Move Breakdown

MUSCLES TO STRENGTHEN

- Glute Med
- Abductors
- Trunk control (abs, obliques etc.)
- Shoulder girdle and Scapulae stabilisers (Trapezius, Serratus Anterior)

MUSCLES TO STRETCH

- Hip Flexors
- Side (obliques)
- Hip adductors

WARNING

- Ensure you roll your shoulders back and don't hang out of your joint, keep your muscles engaged.
- Step into moves- jumping in them uses the force of gravity against you- you come down faster and are more likely to bruise from banging the pole.

STEPS

Step 1: Roll your shoulder back... Outside hand up on the pole, palm facing the direction you are going (behind you)
Step 2: Inside hand wraps around the pole at shoulder height
Step 3: Draw a circle going behind you with your outside leg
Step 4: Lift your inside toe pointing it to your back knee and spin.

Spinning this one to the floor is a great self check aid. you can see where your legs land on the floor, what shape do they make? Do you need to lift more through your obliques and abductors to create a more flat image?

REGRESSIONS

- Backwards Knees
- Seated leg lifts (in spiral position)

PROGRESSIONS

- Play with momentum- walk into it...
- Experiment with smooth dismounts.
- Pirouette or False Step around into Backwards Spiral.

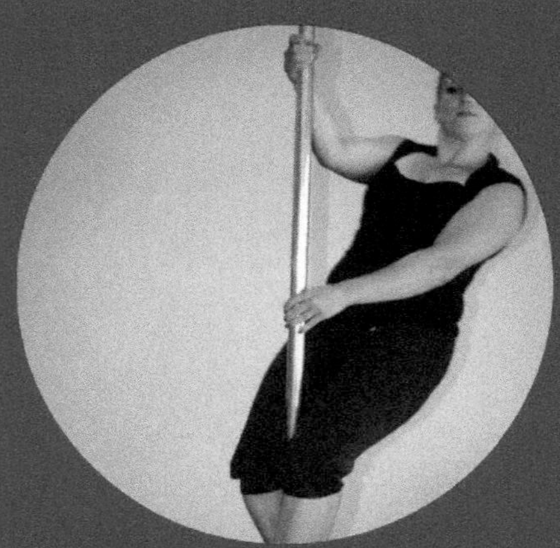

RAPTURE Arts

FIREMAN TO POLE STAND

Rapture Arts Adventures- Pole Move Preparation

Off the Pole

MUSCLES TO STRENGTHEN

- Hip flexors
- Quadriceps
- Adductors
- Shoulder girdle and Scapulae Stabilizers (Trapezius, Serratus Anterior)
- Rotator Cuff (Teres Minor, Infraspinatus)
- Pelvic Floor
- All core (Abdominals and Spine)

CONDITIONING

- Squatting against a wall with ball between legs
- Lunges
- Stepping Lunges
- Step ups
- Prone Shoulder Shrugs
- Prone Shoulder Shrugs with arm lift
- Push Ups against the wall
- Hand conditioning - finger flicks, open and close hand, spread fingers wide and together etc.

MUSCLES TO STRETCH

- Glutes
- Hamstrings
- Triceps
- Latissimus Dorsi
- Pectorals

STRETCH OPTIONS

- Glute stretch (laying down figure 4)
- Standing Hamstring stretch
- Bilateral seated forward bend (pike stretch)
- All grip arm/chest/back/shoulder/neck stretches as per normal warm up and safe practice

*This document is just to serve as a guide and reminder. Posture and alignment is integral. All moves must be performed under professional guidance to ensure correct technique.

RAPTURE Arts

FIREMAN TO POLE STAND

Rapture Arts Adventures- Pole Move Breakdown

MUSCLES TO STRENGTHEN

- Hip flexors
- Quadriceps
- Adductors
- Shoulder girdle and Scapulae stabilisers (Trapezius, Serratus Anterior)
- Core muscles (theres a few there!)

MUSCLES TO STRETCH

- Glutes
- Hamstrings
- Triceps
- Latissimus Dorsi
- Pectorals

WARNING

- Ensure you roll your shoulders back and don't hang out of your joint
- Actively pull with your top arm or you will get a pain in your lower forearm
- Place limbs onto pole to avoid bruising
- Step into moves-not jump

STEPS

Step 1: Inside hand up, palm facing the direction you are going... roll the shoulder back

Step 2: Outside hand across body holding on at chest height

Step 3: Step on inside leg to bring outside leg in front of pole (knee one side, ankle the other) all of the skin of the calf on the pole

Step 4: Tap the other leg to the back of the pole (knee one side, ankle other- so that one knee is on each side of the pole) again as much skin as you can get on the pole.. and start to spin

Step 5: Squeeze legs together on pole

Step 6: Hips up 45 degrees to stand

Step 7: Optional bottom hand up

REGRESSIONS

- Pole lifts, standing or on knees, lifting body off ground if possible
- Basic and Split Grip Fireman
- Straddle, Pike and other abdominally strong spins

PROGRESSIONS

- Play with momentum- walk into it...
- Experiment with smooth dismounts
- You can add in hair flicks or other gestures
- Basic Climb

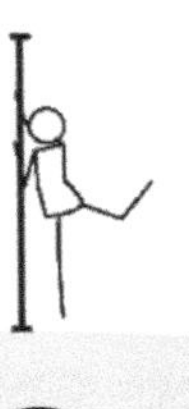

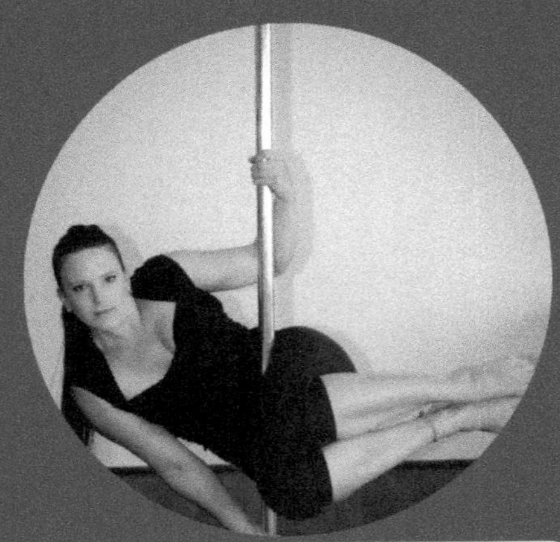

RAPTURE Arts

BASIC CRADLE

Rapture Arts Adventures- Pole Move Preparation

Off the Pole

MUSCLES TO STRENGTHEN

- Bicep
- Shoulder girdle and Scapulae Stabilizers (Trapezius, Serratus Anterior)
- Latissimus Dorsi
- Abdominals and trunk control,
- Elbow stability muscles (if hyper extensive in the elbows)

CONDITIONING

- Modified Clam
- Standing hip adduction with resistance band
- Plank
- Side Plank
- Side plank with leg lift
- Bicep Curls
- Abdominal Crunches
- Abdominal Crunches with twist

GRIP CONDITIONING

- Prone Shoulder Shrugs
- Prone Shoulder Shrugs with arm lift
- Push Ups against the wall
- Potential additions to prevent hyper extending elbows
- Hand conditioning - finger flicks, open and close hand, spread fingers wide and together etc.

MUSCLES TO STRETCH

- Glute Med
- Pectorals
- Obliques

STRETCH OPTIONS

- Pectorals
- All grip arm/chest/back/shoulder/neck stretches as per normal warm up and safe practice

*This document is just to serve as a guide and reminder. Posture and alignment is integral. All moves must be performed under professional guidance to ensure correct technique.

RAPTURE Arts

BASIC CRADLE

Rapture Arts Adventures- Pole Move Breakdown

MUSCLES TO STRENGTHEN

- Bicep
- Shoulder girdle and Scapulae stabilisers (Trapezius, Serratus Anterior)
- Latissimus Dorsi
- Abdominals and trunk control
- Elbow stability muscles (if hyper extensive in the elbows)

STEPS

Step 1: Outside hand across at shoulder height
Step 2: Bring chest to other side of pole
Step 3: Inside hand down to create your triangle grip, finger pointing down the pole
Step 4: Inside leg up, nice and close in hip pocket
Step 5: Outside leg stacks on top to join it
Step 6: Reverse out of it- control legs first then arms

MUSCLES TO STRETCH

- Glute Med
- Pectorals
- Obliques

REGRESSIONS

- Pole lifts, standing or on knees, lifting body off ground if possible
- Straddle Spin
- Peter Pan
- Chair Spin
- Basic Teddy
- Windmill

WARNING

- Ensure you roll your shoulders back and don't hang out of your joint.
- Actively pull with your top arm or you will get a pain in your lower forearm
- Place limbs on to pole to avoid bruising
- Step into moves-not jump

PROGRESSIONS

- Play with momentum- walk into it...
- Experiment with smooth dismounts
- You can extend the top leg
- Jamilla

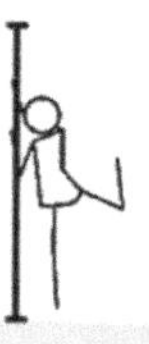

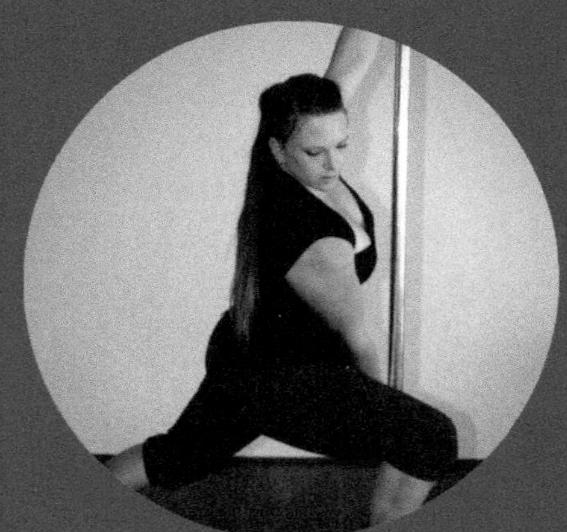

RAPTURE Arts

PETER PAN SPIN

Rapture Arts Adventures- Pole Move Preparation

Off the Pole

MUSCLES TO STREGNTHEN

- Hip Flexors
- Quadriceps
- Trunk extensors (erector spinae)
- Glute max
- Shoulder girdle and Scapulae Stabilizers (Trapezius, Serratus Anterior)
- Pelvic Floor
- All core (Abdominals and Spine)
- Forearm flexors
- Elbow stability muscles (if hyper extensive in the elbows)

CONDITIONING

- Bridging
- 4 point kneeling, leg lifts
- Prone Leg Lift
- Planks - Front and Side

GRIP CONDITIONING

- Prone Shoulder Shrugs
- Prone Shoulder Shrugs with arm lift
- Push Ups against the wall
- Potential conditioning to stop hyper extension of the elbow
- Hand conditioning - finger flicks, open and close hand, spread fingers wide and together etc.

MUSCLES TO STRETCH

- Glutes,
- Hip Flexors
- Rectus Femoris

STRETCH OPTIONS

- Thomas Test Stretch
- Kneeling Hip Flexor Stretch (raise same arm as back leg to point to sky)
- All grip arm/chest/back/shoulder/neck stretches as per normal warm up and safe practice

*This document is just to serve as a guide and reminder. Posture and alignment is integral. All moves must be performed under professional guidance to ensure correct technique.

RAPTURE Arts

PETER PAN SPIN

Rapture Arts Adventures- Pole Move Breakdown

MUSCLES TO STRENGTHEN

- Hip Flexors
- Quadriceps
- Trunk extensors (erector spinae)
- Glute max
- Shoulder girdle and Scapulae stabilisers (Trapezius, Serratus Anterior)
- Abdominals (and the rest of the core),
- Forearm flexors
- Elbow stability muscles (if hyper extensive in the elbows)

MUSCLES TO STRETCH

- Glutes,
- Hip Flexors
- Rectus Femoris

WARNING

- Ensure you roll your shoulders back and don't hang out of your joint.
- Actively pull with your top arm or you will get a pain in your lower forearm
- Place limbs onto pole to avoid bruising
- Step into moves-not jump.

STEPS

Step 1: Roll your shoulder back... Inside hand up, palm facing the direction you are going

Step 2: Place your outside hand on the pole, in split grip position; with your finger pointing down the pole

Step 3: Outside knee comes up nice and high (like a trotting pony)

Step 4: Push off inside leg to straighten and spin.

REGRESSIONS

- Pole lifts, standing or on knees, lifting body off ground if possible
- Shoulder Shrug lifts
- Stag legs in Peter Pan
- Pike Spin
- Straddle Spin

PROGRESSIONS

- Play with momentum- walk into it...
- Experiment with smooth dismounts.

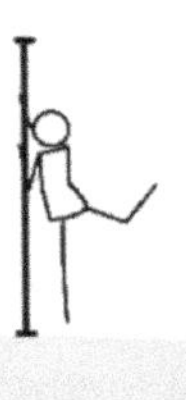

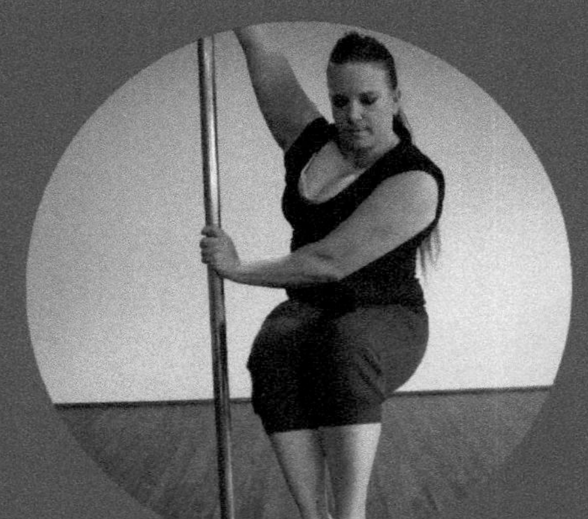

RAPTURE Arts

CHAIR SPIN

Rapture Arts Adventures- Pole Move Preparation

Off the Pole

MUSCLES TO STRENGTHEN

- Obliques
- Hip Flexors
- Shoulder girdle and Scapulae Stabilizers (Trapezius, Serratus Anterior)
- Rotator Cuff (Teres Minor, Infraspinatus)
- Pelvic Floor
- All core (Abdominals and Spine)

CONDITIONING

- Side Planks (can be on knee and elbow)
- Side plank with Arm Peel (top arm comes in front and under torso, then back up to sky)
- Hip Flexor - standing with resistance band

GRIP CONDITIONING

- Prone Shoulder Shrugs
- Prone Shoulder Shrugs with arm lift
- Push Ups against the wall
- Hand conditioning - finger flicks, open and close hand, spread fingers wide and together etc.

MUSCLES TO STRETCH

- Glutes
- Hip Flexors
- Lower Back/Lumbar

STRETCH OPTIONS

- Glute stretch (laying figure 4)
- Kneeling Hip flexor stretch
- Childs pose
- All grip arm/chest/back/shoulder/neck stretches as per normal warm up and safe practice.

*This document is just to serve as a guide and reminder. Posture and alignment is integral. All moves must be performed under professional guidance to ensure correct technique.

RAPTURE Arts

CHAIR SPIN

Rapture Arts Adventures- Pole Move Breakdown

MUSCLES TO STRENGTHEN

- Obliques
- Hip Flexors
- Shoulder girdle and Scapulae stabilisers (Trapezius, Serratus Anterior)
- Rotator Cuff (Teres Minor, Infraspinatus)
- Abdominals (and the rest of the core)

MUSCLES TO STRETCH

- Glutes,
- Hip Flexors
- Lower Back/Lumbar

WARNING

- Ensure you roll your shoulders back and don't hang out of your joint, keep your muscles engaged.
- Place limbs on to pole to avoid bruising
- Step into moves-not jump

STEPS

Step 1: Roll your shoulder back... Inside hand up, palm facing the direction you are going.

Step 2: Outside hand comes across in a Basic Grip Position.

Step 3: Inside knee comes up nice and high.

Step 4: Push off outside leg and bring your knees up and together like you are on a chair - bringing inside knee up first stops the speed wobble until your abs strengthen.

Step 5: As your spin slows, you can step and walk out of it

REGRESSIONS

- Pole lifts, standing or on knees, lifting body off ground if possible
- Shoulder Shrug lifts
- Peter Pan Spin

PROGRESSIONS

- Play with momentum- walk into it...
- Experiment with smooth dismounts
- Paddle/lightly kick legs

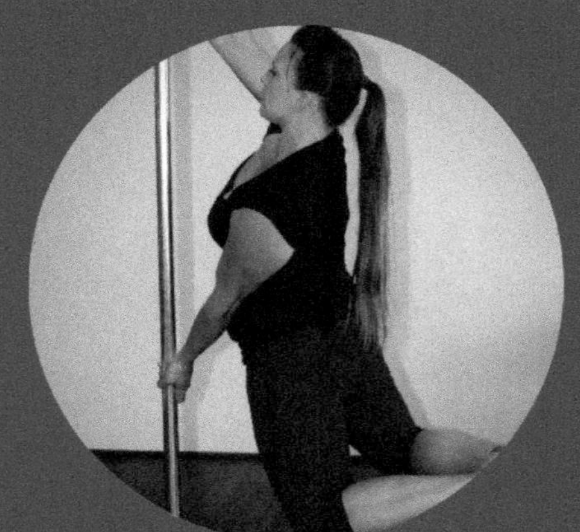

RAPTURE Arts

CAROUSEL SPIN

Rapture Arts Adventures- Pole Move Preparation

Off the Pole

MUSCLES TO STRENGTHEN

- Hip Flexors
- Shoulder girdle and Scapulae Stabilizers (Trapezius, Serratus Anterior)
- Pelvic Floor
- All core (Abdominals and Spine)
- Forearm flexors
- Elbow stability muscles (if hyper extensive in the elbows)

CONDITIONING

- Hamstring Curls
- 4 point kneeling leg lift
- Prone leg lift
- Front Plank

GRIP CONDITIONING

- Prone Shoulder Shrugs
- Prone Shoulder Shrugs with arm lift
- Push Ups against the wall
- Potential conditioning to stop hyper extension of the elbow
- Hand conditioning - finger flicks, open and close hand, spread fingers wide and together etc.

MUSCLES TO STRETCH

- Glutes
- Hip Flexors
- Lower Back/Lumbar

STRETCH OPTIONS

- Kneeling Hip Flexor Stretch (raise same arm as back leg to point to sky)
- Knee Wobble (actually called the Leaning Camel)
- All grip arm/chest/back/shoulder/neck stretches as per normal warm up and safe practice

*This document is just to serve as a guide and reminder. Posture and alignment is integral. All moves must be performed under professional guidance to ensure correct technique.

RAPTURE Arts

CAROUSEL SPIN

Rapture Arts Adventures- Pole Move Breakdown

MUSCLES TO STRENGTHEN

- Hip Flexors
- Shoulder girdle and Scapulae stabilisers (Trapezius, Serratus Anterior)
- Abdominals (and core muscles)
- Forearm flexors
- Elbow stability muscles (if hyper extensive in the elbows)

MUSCLES TO STRETCH

- Glutes,
- Hip Flexors
- Lower Back/Lumbar

WARNING

- Ensure you roll your shoulders back and don't hang out of your joint
- Actively pull with your top arm or you will get a pain in your lower forearm
- Place limbs on to pole to avoid bruising
- Step into moves-not jump.

*Guide Only- does not replace professional training or tuition

STEPS

Step 1: Roll your shoulder back... Inside hand up, palm facing the direction you are going;
Step 2: Step on your inside leg and pivot to face the pole.
Step 3: Place your outside hand on the pole, with your finger pointing down the pole.
Step 4: Bring your outside leg around, bent at the knee as you pivot, leaving it there.... Pull with your top arm, push with your bottom arm...
Step 5: Push off the inside leg as you bend it, (pointing toes together if you wish)

REGRESSIONS

- Pole lifts, standing or on knees, lifting body off ground if possible
- Shoulder Shrug lifts
- Straddle Spin
- Peter Pan
- Chair Spin

PROGRESSIONS

- Play with momentum- walk into it...
- Experiment with smooth dismounts
- You can do a straight legged variation

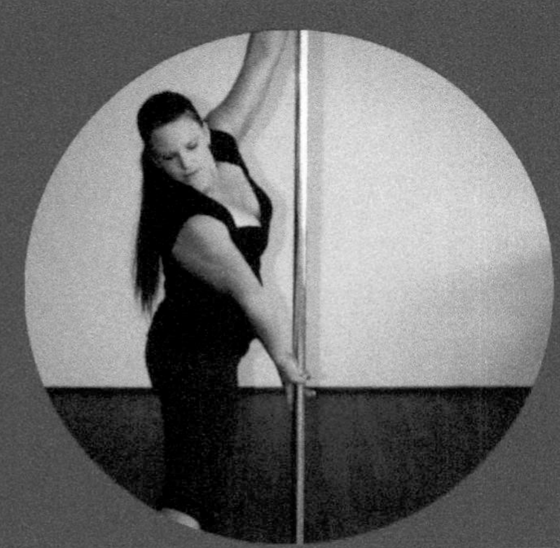

RAPTURE *Arts*

POLE SLIDE

Rapture Arts Adventures- Pole Move Preparation

Off the Pole

MUSCLES TO STRENGTHEN

- Hip Flexors
- Shoulder girdle and Scapulae Stabilizers (Trapezius, Serratus Anterior)
- Pelvic Floor
- All core (Abdominals and Spine)
- Quadriceps
- Forearm flexors
- Elbow stability muscles (if hyper extensive in the elbows)

CONDITIONING

- Abdominal Crunch
- Plank
- Standing Hip Flexion with resistance band
- Quadriceps (squats)

GRIP CONDITIONING

- Prone Shoulder Shrugs
- Prone Shoulder Shrugs with arm lift
- Push Ups against the wall
- Potential conditioning to stop hyper extension of the elbow
- Hand conditioning - finger flicks, open and close hand, spread fingers wide and together etc.

MUSCLES TO STRETCH

- Hamstrings
- Adductors
- Hip Flexors

STRETCH OPTIONS

- Pigeon Pose
- 1/2 Straddle (one leg bent in)
- Kneeling Hip Flexor Stretch (raise same arm as back leg to point to sky)
- All grip arm/chest/back/shoulder/neck stretches as per normal warm up and safe practice

*This document is just to serve as a guide and reminder. Posture and alignment is integral. All moves must be performed under professional guidance to ensure correct technique.

RAPTURE Arts

POLE SLIDE

Rapture Arts Adventures- Pole Move Breakdown

MUSCLES TO STRENGTHEN

- Hip Flexors
- Shoulder girdle and Scapulae stabilisers (Trapezius, Serratus Anterior)
- Abdominals (and the rest of the core),
- Quadriceps
- Forearm flexors
- Elbow stability muscles (if hyper extensive in the elbows)

MUSCLES TO STRETCH

- Hamstrings
- Adductors
- Hip Flexors

WARNING

- Ensure you roll your shoulders back and don't hang out of your joint
- Actively pull with your top arm or you will get a pain in your lower forearm
- Step into moves-not jump
- Do not perform this move without an instructor, there is a high risk of damage if not performed right

*Guide Only- does not replace professional training or tuition

STEPS

Step 1: Roll your shoulder back... inside hand up

Step 2: Place your outside hand on the pole, with your finger pointing down the pole- push and pull with the shoulders

Step 3: Stagger your legs to the side and start edging them out

Step 4: When your down as far as you can, bend your back leg, and sit your bottom back into Jazz Split

REGRESSIONS

- Pole lifts, standing or on knees, lifting body off ground if possible
- Shoulder Shrug lifts
- Straddle Spin
- Pike Spin
- Martini Spin

PROGRESSIONS

- Play with momentum- walk into it...
- Experiment with smooth dismounts
- Slide to splits
- Slide down pole from up high into it

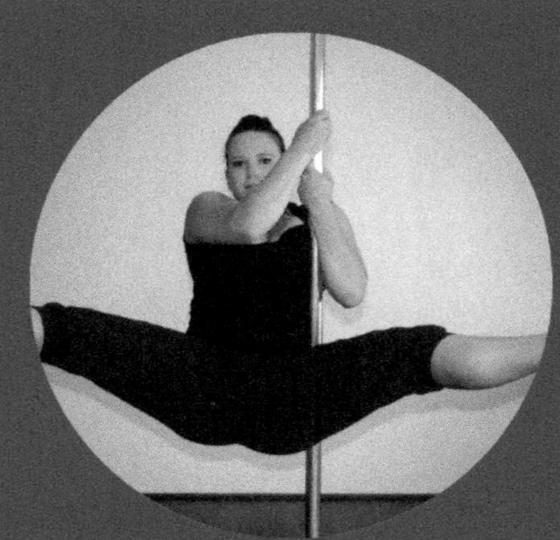

RAPTURE
Arts

BASIC TEDDY

Rapture Arts Adventures- Pole Move Preparation

Off the Pole

MUSCLES TO STRENGTHEN

- Hip Flexors
- Shoulder girdle and Scapulae Stabilizers (Trapezius, Serratus Anterior)
- Rotator Cuff (Teres Minor, Infraspinatus)
- Front line- trunk, abdominals
- Quadriceps

CONDITIONING

- Knee Wobble (actually called the Leaning Camel)
- Abdominal Crunch
- Standing Hip Flexion- with resistance band

GRIP CONDITIONING

- Prone Shoulder Shrugs
- Prone Shoulder Shrugs with arm lift
- Push Ups against the wall
- Rowing
- Shoulder Extension
- Shoulder adduction
- Scapula setting practice
- Hand conditioning - finger flicks, open and close hand, spread fingers wide and together etc.

MUSCLES TO STRETCH

- Hip Adductors
- Hamstrings
- Lower Back/Lumbar

STRETCH OPTIONS

- Straddle Sit- walking hands out to each leg and back; and middle
- All grip arm/chest/back/shoulder/neck stretches as per normal warm up and safe practice

*This document is just to serve as a guide and reminder. Posture and alignment is integral. All moves must be performed under professional guidance to ensure correct technique.

RAPTURE Arts

BASIC TEDDY

Rapture Arts Adventures- Pole Move Breakdown

MUSCLES TO STRENGTHEN

- Hip Flexors
- Shoulder girdle and Scapulae stabilisers (Trapezius, Serratus Anterior)
- Rotator Cuff (Teres Minor, Infraspinatus)
- Front line- trunk, abdominals,
- Quadriceps

MUSCLES TO STRETCH

- Hip Adductors
- Hamstrings
- Lower Back/Lumbar

WARNING

- Ensure you roll your shoulders back and don't hang out of your joint, keeping your muscles engaged.
- Actively pull with your top arm or you will get a pain in your lower forearm
- Place limbs onto pole to avoid bruising
- Step into moves-not jump

*Guide Only- does not replace professional training or tuition

STEPS

Step 1: Inside arm comes around the pole holding the pole at face height, elbow down
Step 2: Outside hand also at face height
Step 3: Squeeze your inside arm on to the pole
Step 4: Bring your hips in front of the pole, resting on the pole
Step 5: Lift into straddle
Step 6: Step your legs down before your arms give in

REGRESSIONS

- Pole lifts, standing or on knees, lifting feet off ground if possible
- Windmill
- Lift into a tuck

PROGRESSIONS

- Play with momentum- walk into it...
- Experiment with smooth dismounts
- Helicopter training drills

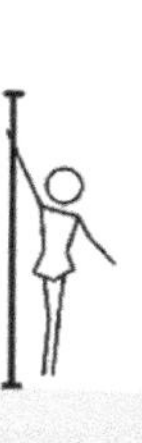

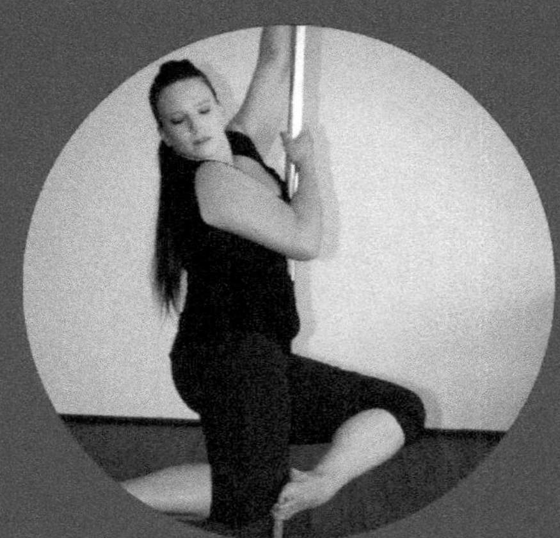

RAPTURE Arts

SWAN

Rapture Arts Adventures- Pole Move Preparation

Off the Pole

MUSCLES TO STRENGTHEN

- Shoulder girdle and Scapulae Stabilizers (Trapezius, Serratus Anterior)
- Rotator Cuff (Teres Minor, Infraspinatus)
- Glute Med
- Abductors
- Trunk control (abs, obliques etc)

CONDITIONING

- Modified Clam
- Standing hip adduction with resistance band
- Plank
- Side Plank
- Side plank with leg lift

GRIP CONDITIONING

- Prone Shoulder Shrugs
- Prone Shoulder Shrugs with arm lift
- Push Ups against the wall
- Hand conditioning - finger flicks, open and close hand, spread fingers wide and together etc.

MUSCLES TO STRETCH

- Hip Adductors
- Hip Flexors
- Obliques

STRETCH OPTIONS

- Kneeling Hip Flexor Stretch (raise same arm as back leg to point to sky)
- All grip arm/chest/back/shoulder/neck stretches as per normal warm up and safe practice

*This document is just to serve as a guide and reminder. Posture and alignment is integral. All moves must be performed under professional guidance to ensure correct technique.

RAPTURE Arts

SWAN

Rapture Arts Adventures- Pole Move Breakdown

MUSCLES TO STRENGTHEN

- Shoulder girdle and Scapulae stabilisers (Trapezius, Serratus Anterior)
- Rotator Cuff (Teres Minor, Infraspinatus)
- Glute Med
- Abductors
- Trunk control (abs, obliques etc)

MUSCLES TO STRETCH

- Hip Adductors
- Hip Flexors
- Obliques

WARNING

- Ensure you roll your shoulders back and don't hang out of your joint
- Actively pull with your top arm or you will get a pain in your lower forearm
- Place limbs onto pole to avoid bruising
- Step into moves-not jump

STEPS

Step 1: Roll your shoulder back... inside hand up, palm facing the direction you are going

Step 2: Outside hand across body holding on at chest height

Step 3: Bring the inside leg up onto the pole, resting it on your upper quad (or hip pocket- where the quad and hip join area)

Step 4: Bring the outside leg up behind you, so that your front toe is pointing to the back knee (fair bit of oblique here to get it flat)

Step 5: Now hold! (or spin on spinning) - you don't want to spin this on a static but you can slide it to the ground

REGRESSIONS

- Pole lifts, standing or on knees, lifting body off ground if possible
- Forwards knees
- Backwards spiral

PROGRESSIONS

- Play with momentum- walk into it...
- Experiment with smooth dismounts

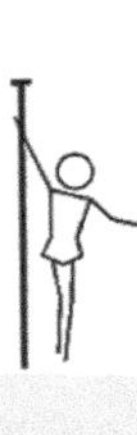

Thank you for letting me be part of your journey.

This journey is your own.

Enjoy it!

(And stay safe.)

xx

Lightning Source UK Ltd.
Milton Keynes UK
UKHW051915090223
416667UK00005B/99